The Wills Eye Drug Guide
Diagnostic and Therapeutic Medications

The Wills Eye Drug Guide
Diagnostic and Therapeutic Medications

Douglas J. Rhee, B.S., M.D.
Resident of Ophthalmology
Wills Eye Hospital
Philadelphia, Pennsylvania

Vincent A. Deramo, B.S., M.D.
Resident of Ophthalmology
Wills Eye Hospital
Philadelphia, Pennsylvania

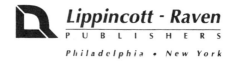

Lippincott - Raven
PUBLISHERS
Philadelphia • New York

Acquisitions Editor: Stuart Freeman
Developmental Editor: David Dritsas
Manufacturing Manager: Tim Reynolds
Production Manager: Robert Pancotti
Production Editor: Christina Zingone
Cover Designer: David Levy
Indexer: Nancy Newman
Compositor: Circle Graphics
Printer: RR Donnelley Crawfordsville

Printed in the United States of America

9 8 7 6 5 4 3 2 1

Library of Congress Cataloging-in-Publication Data
Rhee, Douglas J.
    The Wills eye drug guide : diagnostic and therapeutic medications
    / authors, Douglas J. Rhee, Vincent A. Deramo.
        p.   cm.
    "Intended to complement the Wills eye manual"—Pref.
    Includes bibliographical references and index.
    ISBN 0-7817-1705-1
    1. Ophthalmic drugs—Handbooks, manuals, etc.   I. Deramo,
Vincent A.   II. Wills Eye Hospital (Philadelphia, Pa.)   III. Wills eye
manual.   IV. Title.
    [DNLM: 1. Eye Diseases—drug therapy handbooks.   2. Pharmaceu-
tical Preparations—administration & dosage handbooks.   WW 39 R469w
1998]
RE994.R48   1998
617.7'061—dc21
DNLM/DLC
for Library of Congress   98-9871
                                                                CIP

To my parents, Dennis and Serena Rhee,
in appreciation for their endless love and dedication.
With special gratitude to my mother
whose loving spirit I will always remember.

D.J.R.

To my parents for all their love and support

V.A.D.

Contents

Consultants

WILLS EYE HOSPITAL
900 Walnut Street
Philadelphia, Pennsylvania 19107

Cornea
Christopher J. Rapuano, M.D.

General
Edward A. Jaeger, M.D.
John B. Jeffers, M.D.

Glaucoma
L. Jay Katz, M.D.
Marlene M. Moster, M.D.
George L. Spaeth, M.D.

Infectious Disease
Joselyn Sivalingam, M.D.

Neuro-ophthalmology
Peter J. Savino, M.D.

Oculoplastics
Marlon Maus, M.D.

Pediatrics
Joseph H. Calhoun, M.D.
Leonard B. Nelson, M.D.

Retina
William E. Benson, M.D.
Arunan Sivalingam, M.D.
William Tasman, M.D.
Tamara Vrabec, M.D.

Preface

This pocket reference is designed to assist the eye care professional by providing current information on the ever-increasing number of ocular pharmacotherapeutics. Many different classes of medications are listed, often with pertinent facts. This book presents the usual recommended dose for the medications listed. Clinical judgment should always be used, as all therapy should be tailored to the individual patient. The intent of this manual is to provide therapeutic suggestions once the diagnosis is known. We recommend its use in conjunction with an ophthalmologic reference text. This pocket reference is intended to complement *The Wills Eye Manual: Office & Emergency Room Diagnosis and Treatment of Eye Disease*. More complete listings of all mechanisms, side effects, and drug interactions can be found in the product inserts, the *Physicians' Desk Reference*, and the *Physicians' Desk Reference for Ophthalmology*, and should be consulted.

The Wills Eye Drug Guide

Diagnostic and Therapeutic Medications

1

Antibacterial Agents

TOPICAL ANTIBIOTICS[1]

Drug	Trade	Preparation	Dosage	Notes[a]
bacitracin	N/A[b] AK-Tracin	Soln, 10,000 U/ml Oint, 500 U/g	Q1hr QD–QID	Fortified[c] BC
cefazolin	Ancef	Soln, 5%	Q1hr	Fortified[c]
chloramphenicol	AK-Chlor, Chloromycetin, Chloroptic, Ocu-Chlor	Soln, 0.5%	Q3–6hr	BS, except BC against *Haemophilus influenzae, Neisseria meningitidis, Neisseria gonorrhea, Chlamydia trachomatis* Has been reported to be associated with aplastic anemia
	AK-Chlor, Chloromycetin, Chloroptic, Ocu-Chlor	Oint, 1%	Q3 hr–QHS	
ciprofloxacin	Ciloxan	Soln, 0.3%	Q1/2 hr–QID	Fluoroquinolone, BC; active against *Pseudomonas aeruginosa* and Neisseria species
erythromycin	Ak-mycin, Ilotycin	Oint, 0.5%	QD–QID	BS; active against *N. gonorrhea* and *C. trachomatis*
gentamicin	Garamycin, Genoptic, Gentacidin, Gentak, Ocu-mycin	Soln, 0.3%	Q1–6 hr	Aminoglycoside, BC; active against *P. aeruginosa* and *N. gonorrhea*
	Garamycin, Genoptic,	Oint, 0.3%	QD–TID	

Generic	Trade names	Form, concentration	Dosage	Notes
	Gentacidin, Gentak, Ocu-mycin			
	N/A	Soln, 1.5%	Q1hr	Fortified[c] Periocular use for rosacea **Not for use in the eye**
metronidazole	MetroGel	Gel, 0.75%	BID	
neomycin	Only available in combination medications (see below)			
norfloxacin	Chibroxin	Soln, 0.3%	Q1/2 hr–QID	Fluoroquinolone, BC
ofloxacin	Ocuflox	Soln, 0.3%	Q1/2 hr–QID	Fluoroquinolone, BC
oxytetracycline/polymyxin B	AK-tetra, Terramycin, Terak	Oint, 0.5%/10,000 U	QD–QID	BC
polymyxin B/bacitracin	AK-poly-bac, Polysporin, Polytracin	Oint, 10,000 U/500 U	QD–QID	BC
polymyxin B/neomycin	AK-trol, Statrol	Soln, 16,250 U/0.35%	QID	BC
	AK-trol, Statrol	Oint, 10,000 U/0.35%	QD–QID	
polymyxin B/neomycin/bacitracin	Neotal	Oint, 5,000 U/0.5%/400 U	QD–QID	BC
	AK-Spore, Neosporin, Ocu-spor B	Oint, 10,000 U/0.35%/400 U	QD–QID	
polymyxin B/neomycin/gramicidin	AK-Spore, Neosporin, Ocu-spor G, Polymycin	Soln, 10,000 U/0.35%/0.025%	QID	BC, gramicidin makes cell membrane more permeable
polymyxin B/trimethoprim	Polytrim	Solr, 10,000U/0.1%	QID	BC

Antibacterial Agents

continued

[1]For antibiotic spectrum of topical agents, refer to Appendix 1.

Drug	Trade	Preparation	Dosage	Notes[a]
sulfacetamide	AK-Sulf, Bleph-10, Ophthacet, Ocusulf, Sulf-10, Sulamyd Sodium	Soln, 10%	Q1hr–QID	BS
	Isopto Cetamide	Soln, 15%	Q1hr–QID	
	Isopto Cetamide	Soln, 30%	Q1hr–QID	
	AK-Sulf, Cetamide, Sulamyd Sodium	Oint, 10%	QD–QID	
sulfacetamide/ phenylephrine	Vasosulf	Soln, 15%/0.125%	QD–QID	BS; antibiotic with an alpha agonist
sulfisoxazole	Gantrisin	Soln, 4%	Q1hr–QID	BS
	Gantrisin	Oint, 4%	QD–QID	
tetracycline	Achromycin	Soln, 1%	Q1hr–QID	BS
tobramycin	AKTOB, Defy, Tobrex	Soln, 0.3%	Q1–4hr	Aminoglycoside, BC; active against *P. aeruginosa* and *N. gonorrhea*
	AKTOB, Defy, Tobrex	Oint, 0.3%	QD–TID	Fortified[c]
	Tobrex	Soln, 1.5%	Q1hr	Fortified[c]; **not** for gram-negative coverage
vancomycin	Vancocin	Soln, 5%	Q1hr	

[a]BC, bacteriocidal; BS, bacteriostatic.
[b]N/A, not available.
[c]Fortified medications not commercially available; refer to Appendix 2 for preparation instructions.

ORAL ANTIBIOTICS

Drug	Trade	Dosage	Notes
amoxicillin	Amoxil, Polymox	250–500 mg PO TID	Adult dose
		25–50 mg/kg/day PO in 3 divided doses	Pediatric dose
amoxicillin/clavulanate	Augmentin	250–500 mg PO TID or 875 mg PO BID	Adult dose
		20–40 mg/kg/day PO in 3 divided doses	Pediatric dose
azithromycin	Zithromax	500 mg PO day 1, then 250 mg QD × 4 days	Adult Dose
		1,000 mg PO × 1 dose	Dose for *Chlamydia* urethritis
		5–12 mg/kg/day PO in one dose × 5 days	Pediatric dose
cephalexin	Keflex	250–500 mg PO QID	Adult dose
		25–50 mg/kg/day PO in 4 divided doses	Pediatric dose
cefuroxime axetil	Ceftin	250–500 mg PO BID	Adult dose
		20–30 mg/kg/day PO divided BID	Pediatric dose
ciprofloxacin	Cipro	250–750 mg PO BID	Not for children or during pregnancy
			Not to be taken with antacids
clarithromycin	Biaxin	250–500 mg PO BID	Adult dose
		15 mg/kg/day PO divided BID	Pediatric dose
doxycycline	Vibramycin	100 mg BID	Can be used for ocular rosacea
			Not for children or during pregnancy
erythromycin	E-mycin	250–500 mg PO QID	Adult dose
		30–50 mg/kg/day in 3–4 divided doses	Pediatric dose

continued

Drug	Trade	Dosage	Notes
minocycline	Minocin	100–200 mg PO BID	Not for children or during pregnancy
ofloxacin	Floxin	200–400 mg PO BID	Not for children or during pregnancy
tetracycline	Achromycin	250–500 mg PO QID	Can be used for ocular rosacea Not for children or during pregnancy Not to be taken with food, milk products, or antacids

ANTIBIOTICS FOR SUBCONJUNCTIVAL/INTRAVITREAL INJECTION

Aminoglycosides[2]

	Subconjunctival injection[a]	Intravitreal injection[b]
amikacin	25 mg	0.2–0.4 mg
gentamicin	10–20 mg	0.2–0.4 mg
kanamycin	30 mg	N/A[c]
neomycin	125–250 mg	N/A
tobramycin	10–20 mg	0.1–0.2 mg

[a]Subconjunctival dose should be in a volume of 0.5 ml.
[b]Intravitreal dose should be in a volume of 0.1 ml.
[c]N/A, not available.

[2]All intravitreal injections of aminoglycosides have potential for macular necrosis.

Penicillins

	Subconjunctival injection[a]	Intravitreal injection[b]	Notes
ampicillin	50–150 mg	0.5 mg	Rarely used
carbenicillin	100 mg	0.25–2.0 mg	—
methicillin	50–100 mg	1.0–2.0 mg	—
penicillin G	0.5–1.0 million U	N/A[c]	—
ticarcillin	100 mg	N/A	—

[a]Subconjunctival dose should be in a volume of 0.5 ml.
[b]Intravitreal dose should be in a volume of 0.1 ml.
[c]N/A, not available.

Cephalosporins

	Subconjunctival injection[a]	Intravitreal injection[b]	Notes
cefazolin	100 mg	2.0–2.25 mg	First generation, rarely used
ceftazidime	200 mg	2.25 mg	Third generation

[a]Subconjunctival dose should be in a volume of 0.5 ml.
[b]Intravitreal dose should be in a volume of 0.1 ml.

Others

Drug	Subconjunctival injection[a]	Intravitreal injection[b]	Notes
bacitracin	5,000 U	N/A[c]	—
chloramphenicol	N/A	1.0 mg	Rarely used
clindamycin	15–50 mg	1.0 mg	—
erythromycin	100 mg	0.5 mg	Almost never used
polymyxin B sulfate	100,000 U	N/A	—
vancomycin	25 mg	1.0 mg	—

[a]Subconjunctival dose should be in a volume of 0.5 ml.
[b]Intravitreal dose should be in a volume of 0.1 ml.
[c]N/A, not available.

REGIMENS FOR SPECIFIC ORGANISMS

Syphilis[3]

Notes: 1. Caused by *Treponema pallidum.*
2. Both patient and sexual partners must be evaluated for other sexually transmitted diseases, including HIV.

Early

Primary, secondary, or latent infection less than 1 year.

[3]From *Med Lett* 1995;37:120.

Drug	Dosage
penicillin G benzathine	2.4 million U IM once (may repeat 7 days later in patients with AIDS)
or	
doxycycline	100 mg PO BID × 14 days

Late
Includes isolated anterior uveitis; latent infection more than 1 year's duration; cardiovascular; gumma.

Drug	Dosage
penicillin G benzathine	2.4 million U IM weekly × 3 wk
or	
doxycycline	100 mg PO BID × 4 wk

Neurosyphilis
Includes posterior uveitic involvement.

Note: PCN-allergic patients may need to be desensitized.

Drug	Dosage
penicillin G	2–4 million U IV Q4hr × 10–14 days followed by penicillin G benzathine 2.4 million U IM Q wk × 3 doses

Congenital

Drug	Dosage
penicillin G	50,000 U/kg IM or IV Q 8–12 hr × 10–14 days

Gonococcal Conjunctivitis/Keratitis[4]

Notes:
1. Caused by *Neisseria gonorrhea*
2. Patient's sexual partners must be treated. Both patient and sexual partners must be evaluated for other manifestations of gonorrhea and for other sexually transmitted diseases, including HIV and syphilis.
3. Patients must also be treated for concurrent chlamydial infection, which may be present.
4. In penicillin/cephalosporin-allergic patients, an infectious disease consultation may be needed.
5. All patients should receive warm saline irrigation of fornices.
6. Also administer topical antibiotics:
   - Bacitracin or erythromycin ointment QID (may use ciprofloxacin solution Q2hr (adults only)) for conjunctivitis only.
   - Ciprofloxacin or gentamicin or tobramycin solution Q1hr for **corneal** involvement

[4]From *Med Lett* 1995;37:119.

Drug	Trade	Dosage	Notes
ceftriaxone	Rocephin	1 g IM × 1 dose 25–50 mg/kg IV QD × 7 days 125 mg IM × 1 dose	For adult GC conjunctivitis For child with GC conjunctivitis [a] For **neonatal gonococcal conjunctivitis**; do not use with hyperbilirubinemic neonates
cefotaxime	Claforan	1–2 g IV QD × 3 days 50 mg/kg IV or IM Q8–12hr × 7 days	For adult GC corneal ulcer For **neonatal gonococcal conjunctivitis**

[a]Cullom RD, Chang B, eds. *The Wills eye manual: office and emergency room diagnosis and treatment of eye disease*, 2nd ed. Philadelphia: JB Lippincott Co, 1994.

Chlamydial Inclusion Conjunctivitis or Trachoma

Notes:
1. Duration of treatment is 3 weeks for inclusion conjunctivitis (caused by *Chlamydia trachomatis* Subtypes D–K) and 3 to 6 weeks for trachoma (caused by *C. trachomatis* Subtypes A–C).[5]
2. Diagnosis of inclusion conjunctivitis requires that patient's sexual partners be treated. Both patient and sexual partners must be evaluated for other sexually transmitted diseases, including HIV.
3. Select one ointment **and** one oral agent.

[5]From Frauenfelder F, Roy FH. *Current ocular therapy. 4.* Philadelphia: WB Saunders, 1995:62–63.

Drug	Trade	Dosage	Notes
erythromycin	Ak-mycin, Ilotycin	Oint, 0.5% BID–TID × 3–6 wk	Recommended for **neonatal chlamydial** conjunctivitis
oxytetracycline/ polymyxin B	AK-tetra, Terramycin, Terak	Oint, 0.5%/10,000 U BID–TID × 3–6 wk	Not for children or during pregnancy
sulfacetamide	AK-Sulf, Bleph-10, Cetamide, Sulamyd Sodium	Oint, 10% BID–TID × 3–6 wk	—
plus			
clarithromycin	Biaxin	250–500 mg PO BID × 3–6 wk 15 mg/kg/day PO divided BID × 3–6 wk	Adult dose Pediatric dose
doxycycline	Vibramycin	100 mg PO BID × 3–6 wk	Not for children or during pregnancy
erythromycin	E-mycin	250–500 mg PO QID × 3–6 wk 50 mg/kg/day PO divided QID × 3–6 wk	Adult dose Pediatric dose, recommended for 14 days in **neonatal chlamydial** conjunctivitis
ofloxacin	Floxin	300 mg PO BID × 3–6 wk	Not for children or during pregnancy
tetracycline	Achromycin	250–500 mg PO QID × 3–6 wk	Not for children or during pregnancy

Lyme Disease[6]

Caused by *Borrelia burgdorferi*. If patient has ocular involvement beyond follicular conjunctivitis occurring within the first month of infection, must be considered to have central nervous system (CNS) involvement.

[6]From Sanford JP, Gilbert DN, Sande, MA. *Sanford guide to antimicrobial therapy.* Dallas, Texas: Antimicrobial Therapy, Inc., 1995:38–39.

Stage 1 (Erythema Migrans)

Early (limited to follicular conjunctivitis as above). Select **one** agent and treat for 14 to 21 days (except azithromycin).

Drug	Trade	Dosage	Notes
amoxicillin	Amoxil	500 mg PO TID 20–40 mg/kg/day PO in 3 divided doses	Preferred first-line agent Pediatric dose
azithromycin	Zithromax	500 mg PO QD × 1 day, then 250 mg PO QD × 4 days	—
cefuroxime	Ceftin	500 mg PO BID 20–30 mg/kg/day PO divided BID	Adult dose Pediatric dose (max 1 g/day)
clarithromycin	Biaxin	250–500 mg PO BID 15 mg/kg/day PO divided BID	Adult dose Pediatric dose
doxycycline	Vibramycin	100 mg PO BID	Preferred first-line agent Not for children or during pregnancy
erythromycin	E-mycin	250 mg PO QID 30–50 mg/kg/day in 3–4 divided doses	Adult dose Pediatric dose
tetracycline	Achromycin	250 mg PO QID	Not for children or during pregnancy

Stage 2

Develops in days to months, dissemination of organism to skin, heart, joints, and CNS. Ocular involvement consists of granulomatous anterior uveitis, retinal vasculitis, choroiditis, keratitis, intermediate uveitis, and optic neuritis. Select **one** agent—patient needs systemic work-up to rule out arthritis, which must be treated with ceftriaxone or doxycycline.

Drug	Trade	Dosage	Notes
cefotaxime	Claforan	3.0 g IV Q12h × 21–28 days	—
ceftriaxone	Rocephin	2.0 g IV QD × 21–28 days 50–75 mg/kg/day divided Q 12 hr	Preferred first-line agent Pediatric dose (max 2 g/day)
doxycycline	Vibramycin	100 mg PO BID	Preferred first-line agent Not for children or during pregnancy
penicillin G	—	2–4 million U IV Q4hr × 21–28 days	—

Stage 3

Develops weeks to years following initial infection and is typically characterized by development of arthritis. Ocular involvement includes episcleritis, stromal keratitis, orbital myositis, chronic meningitis, chronic arthritis, adult respiratory distress syndrome.

Drug[a]	Trade	Dosage	Notes
ceftriaxone	Rocephin	2.0 g IV QD × 14–28 days 50–75 mg/kg/day divided Q12hr	Preferred first-line agent Pediatric dose (max 2 g/day)
or			
doxycycline	Vibramycin	100 mg PO BID × 30 days	Not for children or during pregnancy

[a]*Borrelia burgdorferi* in fibroblasts not killed by ceftriaxone; azithromycin and clarithromycin may be drugs of choice (*J Antimicrob Chemother* 1990;25:A–33); however, no comparative clinical studies are available.

REGIMENS FOR SPECIFIC CLINICAL ENTITIES

Blepharitis

Notes: 1. Treated with combination of warm compresses, lid hygiene (using warm wash cloth with baby shampoo to scrub lashes), and artificial tears four to eight times per day, depending on the severity of dry eye symptoms.
2. May supplement with either erythromycin or bacitracin ointment at bedtime.
3. Additionally, may use a combination antibiotic/steroid (e.g., Vasocidin, Blephamide) QID. However, we recommend short duration of treatment and extreme care to monitor for side effects of topical steroids.
4. For severe posterior blepharitis or ocular rosacea, may supplement with an oral agent (see below, Rosacea, Ocular).

Rosacea, Ocular

Select **one** agent, in addition to warm compresses, lid hygiene, and artificial tears. For oral agents, treat for 3 to 6 weeks, then decrease dosing frequency by half (e.g., BID → QD) and continue for several months.

Drug	Trade	Dosage	Notes
doxycycline	Vibramycin	100 mg PO BID	Not for children or during pregnancy
erythromycin	E-mycin	250 mg PO QID	If unable to take doxycycline or tetracycline
metronidazole	MetroGel	Gel, 0.75%, apply BID	Periocular use for rosacea **Not for use in the eye**
tetracycline	Achromycin	250 mg PO QID	Not for children or during pregnancy

Stye/Hordeolum

Notes: 1. Warm compress with massage over the affected area four times per day.
2. Medications are not indicated unless preseptal cellulitis occurs (see below, Preseptal Cellulitis).

Pediculosis

Notes: 1. Caused by *Phthirus pubis*; lice, "crabs."
2. Use antilice lotion and shampoo for nonocular areas: e.g., permethrin 5% (Elimite) or Lindane Shampoo 1%.
3. Additionally, lice and nits (eggs) may be removed from lids/lashes with fine forceps at the slit lamp.
4. All sexual partners need to be examined; instruct the patient to wash all linens and sheets.
5. Physostigmine interferes with the organism's respiratory function, but has significant ocular side effects and is rarely used.

Drug	Trade	Dosage	Notes
Any bland ophthalmic ointment (bacitracin, erythromycin)		TID for 10 days	(Smothers lice and nits)
or			
physostigmine	Eserine	Oint, 0.25% (see notes)	Two applications to lids 1 wk apart; has significant ocular side effects; rarely used

Conjunctivitis

Viral

Antibacterial medications are not indicated in most viral conjunctivitis unless significant corneal epithelial damage has occurred, to prevent secondary bacterial infections. For symptomatic improvement, consider artificial tears, ocular decongestant/antihistamine (e.g., naphazoline/pheiramine), and cool compresses.

Bacterial

If clinically suspect bacterial conjunctivitis, Gram stain and culture appropriately and start on a broad-spectrum topical agent (e.g., polymyxin/trimethoprim, ciprofloxacin, ofloxacin four to six times per day). Certain etiologies (e.g., *N. gonorrhea*) are relative emergencies and should be managed according to specific regimens.

Neonatal

Most commonly caused by *C. trachomatis, Streptococcus viridans, Staphylococcus aureus, Haemophilus influenzae,* group B *Streptococcus, Moraxella catarrhalis,* or *Neisseria gonorrhea.* Treatment is guided by Gram stain (which should be performed immediately to identify *N. gonorrhea*) and culture results. *N. gonorrhea* and *C. trachomatis* have specific regimens as described (see conjunctivitis, neonatal, in Subject Index). If not gonococcal or chlamydial, may use erythromycin ointment Q4–6hr as only initial treatment.

Canaliculitis

Notes: 1. Etiologies include *Actinomyces israelii* (most common), viruses, chlamydia, fungi, and other bacteria.
2. Surgical removal of offending agent is the most important aspect of treatment. Evaluate drainage system for obstruction, attempt to remove concretions, and obtain smears and cultures of any material expressed.
3. Consider irrigation of canaliculus with penicillin G solution 100,000 U/ml, repeat as necessary; irrigation should be performed in upright position so drainage is out nose rather than nasopharynx.
4. Consider tetracycline 250 mg PO QID (not for use in children or during pregnancy) or Bactrim DS one tab PO BID, for bacterial etiologies.
5. If fungus is recovered, irrigate with nystatin 1:20,000 U/ml in addition to topical nystatin drops TID.
6. If herpes is found, treat with trifluridine 1% drops five time per day for several weeks.
7. Warm compresses QID.

Dacryocystitis

Notes: 1. All patients receive topical polymyxin/trimethoprim (Polytrim) QID in addition to systemic antibiotics.
2. All patients receive warm compresses QID.

3. May require surgical incision and drainage if abscess is present.
4. May require surgical reconstruction of nasolacrimal drainage system (e.g., Dacryocystorhinostomy [DCR]) 1 to 4 weeks after acute inflammation is resolved.
5. Fungal etiologies usually have a more subacute or chronic presentation; *Aspergillus* is most common fungal cause (see **Aspergillosis**).
6. Pediatric consultation is recommended in children.

Afebrile, Mild Case, Systemically Well, Reliable Patient/Parent
Select **one** agent with daily follow-up.

Drug	Trade	Dosage	Notes
amoxicillin/clavulanate	Augmentin	500 mg PO TID or 875 mg PO BID	Adult dose
		20–40 mg/kg/day PO in 3 divided doses	Pediatric dose
cefaclor	Ceclor	250 mg PO TID	Adult dose
		20–40 mg/kg/day PO in 3 divided doses	Pediatric dose
cephalexin	Keflex	500 mg PO QID	Adult dose
		25–50 mg/kg/day PO in 4 divided doses	Pediatric dose

Febrile, Moderate–Severe Case, Acutely ill, Unreliable parent
Hospitalize and select **one** agent.

Drug	Trade	Dosage	Notes
cefazolin	Ancef	1 g IV Q8hr 25–50 mg/kg/day IV in 3 divided doses	Adult dose Pediatric dose
cefuroxime	Zinacef	1.5 g IV Q8hr 75–100 mg/kg/day IV in 3 divided doses	Adult dose Pediatric dose

Dacryoadenitis—Bacterial

Notes:
1. Other causes of lacrimal gland masses include inflammatory, neoplastic, and viral causes. Refer to the *Wills Eye Manual*[7] for complete discussion on evaluation of nonbacterial treatment.
2. Computed tomography (CT) scan of orbit and brain to rule out abscess formation which may require surgical incision and drainage.
3. Pediatric consultation is recommended in children.

Mild

Select **one** agent with daily follow-up.

Drug	Trade	Dosage	Notes
amoxicillin/clavulanate	Augmentin	250–500 mg PO TID or 875 mg PO BID 20–40 mg/kg/day in 3 divided doses	Adult dose Pediatric dose
cephalexin	Keflex	250–500 mg PO QID 25–50 mg/kg/day in 4 divided doses	Adult dose Pediatric dose

[7]From Cullom RD, Chang B, eds. *The Wills eye manual: office and emergency room diagnosis and treatment of eye disease,* 2nd ed. Philadelphia: JB Lippincott Co, 1994.

Moderate to Severe
Hospitalize and select **one** agent.

Drug	Trade	Dosage	Notes
ticarcillin/clavulanate	Timentin	3.1 g IV Q4–6hr 200 mg/kg/day in 4 divided doses	Adult dose Pediatric dose above age 12 mo
cefazolin	Ancef	1 g IV Q8hr 50–100 mg/kg/day IV in 3 divided doses	Adult dose Pediatric dose over 1 mo of age (max adult dose 4–6 g/day)

Preseptal Cellulitis

Mild Case, Patient Older than 5 Years of Age, Afebrile, Systemically Well, Reliable Patient / Parent
Select **one** agent with daily follow-up and treat for 10 days.

Drug	Trade	Dosage	Notes
amoxicillin/clavulanate	Augmentin	250–500 mg PO TID or 875 PO BID 20–40 mg/kg/day PO in 3 divided doses	Adult dose Pediatric dose
cefaclor	Ceclor	250–500 mg PO TID 20–40 mg/kg/day PO in 3 divided doses	Adult dose Pediatric dose
cephalexin	Keflex	250–500 mg PO QID 25–50 mg/kg/day in 4 divided doses	Adult dose Pediatric dose

clarithromycin	Biaxin	250–500 mg PO BID — Adult dose
		15 mg/kg/day PO divided BID — Pediatric dose
erythromycin	E-mycin	250–500 mg PO QID — Adult dose
		30–50 mg/kg/day PO in 3–4 divided doses — Pediatric dose
trimethoprim/	Bactrim	One double strength tablet PO BID — Adult dose
sulfamethoxazole		8–12 mg/kg/day TMX and 40–60 mg/kg/day SMX PO in 2 divided doses — Pediatric dose

Moderate–Severe Preseptal Cellulitis or Child Younger than 5 Years of Age

Hospitalize and give **Both** agents.

Notes: 1. Patient may be switched to oral therapy after significant improvement has occurred; total duration of systemic therapy should be for 10 to 14 days.

2. Children under 5 years old must receive complete physical examination to rule out concurrent otitis media, sinusitis, and bacteremia. Pediatric consultation is recommended.

Drug	Trade	Dosage	Notes
ceftriaxone	Rocephin	1–2 g IV Q12hr	Adult dose
		100 mg/kg/day IV in 2 divided doses	Pediatric dose
and			

continued

			Adult dose[a]
vancomycin	Vancocin	0.5–1 g IV Q12hr	Adult dose[a]
		40 mg/kg/day IV in 3–4 divided doses	Pediatric dose[a]
		15 mg/kg load, maintenance dose 10 mg/kg BID–TID	Neonatal dose[a]

[a]Follow peak and trough drug levels; dose must be adjusted in renal failure.

Orbital Cellulitis—Bacterial

Children

Give **both** agents; pediatric consultation is recommended.

Drug	Trade	Dosage	Notes
ceftriaxone and	Rocephin	100 mg/kg/day IV in 2 divided doses	—
vancomycin	Vancocin	40 mg/kg/day IV in 3–4 divided doses	Pediatric dose[a]
		15 mg/kg load, maintenance dose 10 mg/kg BID–TID	Neonatal dose[a]

[a]Follow peak and trough drug levels; dose must be adjusted in renal failure.

Adults

Give either ampicillin/sulbactam alone or ceftriaxone plus vancomycin.

Drug	Trade	Dosage	Notes
ampicillin/sulbactam	Unasyn	1.5–3.0 g IV Q6hr × 7 days	—
ceftriaxone	Rocephin	1–2 g IV Q12hr × 7 days	Continue oral antibiotics on discharge
vancomycin	Vancocin	1 g IV Q12hr × 7 days[a]	Continue oral antibiotics on discharge

[a]Follow peak and trough drug levels; dose must be adjusted in renal failure.

Notes:
1. If highly suspect adults with anaerobic infections, consider adding metronidazole 15 mg/kg IV load, then 7.5 mg/kg IV Q6hr, or clindamycin 600 mg IV Q8hr (ampicillin/sulbactam alone has adequate anaerobic coverage).
2. If adult patient is allergic to penicillin/cephalosporin, may use vancomycin plus gentamicin 2.0 mg/kg IV loading dose, then 1 mg/kg IV Q8hr **or** clindamycin 600 mg IV Q8hr plus gentamicin.
3. If no improvement, suspect abscess or resistant organism.

Ruptured Globe (Including Full Thickness Corneal Laceration)

Notes:
1. On presentation, shield eye without contact to globe and keep patient NPO.
2. Treatment is prompt surgical exploration and repair.
3. Admit and give systemic antibiotics—give **two** (i.e., give gentamicin or ciprofloxacin with either vancomycin or cefazolin).
4. Consider CT scan to rule out intraocular and/or intraorbital foreign body
5. If no endophthalmitis develops after 3 days of IV therapy, may change to oral ciprofloxacin 250–750 mg BID. Ciprofloxacin not for children or during pregnancy.
6. If tetanus immunization is not up to date, give tetanus toxoid 0.5 ml IM.
7. If endophthalmitis does develop, see **Endophthalmitis—traumatic.**

Drug	Trade	Dosage	Notes
vancomycin	Vancocin	1 g IV Q12hr	Adult dose[a]
		40 mg/kg/day IV in 2–4 divided doses	Pediatric dose[a]
or		15 mg/kg load, maintenance dose 10 mg/kg BID–TID	Neonatal dose[a]
cefazolin	Ancef	1 g IV Q8hr	Adult dose
		25–50 mg/kg/day IV in 3 divided doses	Pediatric dose
plus			
ciprofloxacin	Cipro	200–400 mg IV BID	Not for children or during pregnancy
or			
gentamicin	Garamycin	2.0 mg/kg IV load, then 1 mg/kg IV Q8hr maintenance	Adult dose[a]
		2.0 mg/kg IV Q8hr	Pediatric dose[a]

Blebitis

Most commonly associated with *Streptococcus* species and *H. influenzae.*

Suspected Bleb Infection, but No Anterior Chamber or Vitreal Involvement

Notes: 1. Consider culturing bleb for diagnostic purposes.
2. Select antibiotic regimen (use ofloxacin alone or both tobramycin and vancomycin).

Drug	Trade	Preparation	Dosage	Notes
ofloxacin	Ocuflox	Soln, 0.3%	Q1hr	Mild case
or				
tobramycin (fortified)[a]	Tobrex	Soln, 1.5%	Q1hr	Moderate–severe case
and				
vancomycin (fortified)[a]	Vancocin	Soln, 5%	Q1hr	Moderate–severe case

[a]Fortified medications not commercially available, refer to Appendix 2 for preparation instructions.

3. Reevaluate after 12 to 24 hours, and if there is improvement, consider adding steroid to prevent loss of bleb.

Drug	Trade	Preparation	Dosage
prednisolone acetate	Pred Forte, Econopred Plus	Susp, 1%	QID

Suspected Bleb Infection with Anterior Chamber, but No Vitreal Involvement

Notes: 1. Consider culturing bleb and/or performing anterior chamber tap for diagnostic purposes.
2. Begin antibiotics immediately; use both drops alternating every half hour; consider admission to hospital.

Drug	Trade	Preparation	Dosage
tobramycin (fortified)[a] and	Tobrex	Soln, 1.5%	Q1hr
vancomycin (fortified)[a]	Vancocin	Soln, 5%	Q1hr

[a]Fortified medications not commercially available; refer to Appendix 2 for preparation instructions.

3. Reevaluate after 12 to 24 hours, and if there is improvement, consider adding steroid to prevent loss of bleb.

Drug	Trade	Preparation	Dosage
prednisolone acetate	Pred Forte, Econopred Plus	Susp, 1%	Q2hr

Suspected Bleb Infection with Anterior Chamber and Vitreal Involvement
See below, Endophthalmitis.

Endophthalmitis

Postoperative—Acute (Less than 1 Week)

Notes: 1. Most common organism encountered is *Staphylococcus epidermidis*; others include *S. aureus, Streptococcus species, Serratia marcescens, Proteus* species, and *Pseudomonas* species).

2. Intravitreal antibiotics are the treatment of choice, combined with topical antibiotics; the benefit of subconjunctival antibiotics is controversial at this time and they are not frequently used (see below for dosing).

3. Immediate pars plana vitrectomy is benefical if visual acuity on presentation is light perception or worse.[8]

[8]From *Arch Ophthalmol* 1995;113:1479–1496.

4. Often combined with topical, subconjunctival, and/or intravitreal steroids since fungi are unlikely in the early postoperative setting. Use topical prednisolone acetate 1% Q1hr and subconjunctival triamcinolone 40 mg at the time of vitrectomy. Intravitreal dexamethasone 0.4 mg at time of surgery is at surgeon's discretion.

5. Topical atropine 1% TID is also given for cycloplegia.

TOPICAL. Combination of fortified aminoglycoside with either fortified cefazolin or vancomycin.

Drug[a]	Dosage
fortified cefazolin or fortified vancomycin	Q1hr (alternate drops every 30 min)
plus	
fortified gentamicin or fortified tobramycin	Q1hr (alternate drops every 30 min)

[a]Fortified medications not commercially available; refer to Appendix 2 for preparation instructions.

INTRAVITREAL

Notes: 1. Can be reinjected if the vitreous is not clearing.
2. Ceftazidime is alternative agent for gram-negative coverage in bacterial endophthalmitis.[9]

Drug	Dosage		Drug	Dosage
amikacin	0.2–0.4 mg in 0.1 ml	or	ceftazidime	2.25 mg in 0.1 ml
plus				
vancomycin	1.0 mg in 0.1 ml (clindamycin 1 mg in 0.1 ml may be used in place of vancomycin)			

[9]From *Surv Ophthalmol* 1997;41:395–401.

SUBCONJUNCTIVAL

Drug	Dosage		Drug	Dosage
ceftazidime	100 mg in 0.5 ml	and	vancomycin	25–50 mg in 0.5 ml

Postoperative—Delayed (Longer than 1 Week)

Notes:
1. Begin treatment as with Postoperative—Acute, except do **Not** use steroids if fungal etiology is suspected.
2. Immediate pars plana vitrectomy is beneficial if visual acuity on presentation is light perception or worse up to 6 weeks following surgery.[10] Benefit beyond 6 weeks is not known.
3. If *Propionibacterium acnes* infection is suspected (usually from 2 months to several years following cataract surgery with granulomatous keratic precipitates, anterior uveitis, vitritis, and white plaques in capsular bag (often with retained lens material)), intravitreal vancomycin combined with local debridement/removal of intracapsular plaques may be sufficient.
4. If mild *S. epidermidis* is isolated, intraocular vancomycin alone may be sufficient.
5. If fungus is suspected (usually begins approximately 3 months after surgery—*Candida* is most commonly encountered organism), consider amphotericin B 5–10 µg at time of vitrectomy.
6. If fungus is identified on Gram stain, Giemsa, or Calcofluor white, then use combination of topical and systemic antifungal medications. Use topical natamycin 5% Q1hr and flucytosine 37.5 mg/kg PO Q6hr until specific organism is known. Role of systemic amphotericin B and fluconazole is unclear.
7. Consider miconazole 10 mg in 1 ml subconjunctivally.

[10]From *Arch Opthalmol* 1995;113:1479–1496.

Traumatic

Notes:

1. Begin treatment as with Postoperative—Acute, except do **not** use steroids, and therapeutic benefit of pars plana vitrectomy (PPV) is unknown for this type of endophthalmitis. However, PPV offers the theoretical benefit of reducing infectious load and providing sufficient material for diagnostic culture and pathology.

2. Intravitreal amikacin 0.4 mg in 0.1 ml or ceftriaxone 2 mg in 0.1 ml along with intravitreal vancomycin 1.0 mg in 0.1 ml should be given. May repeat Q2–3days. (Clindamycin 1 mg in 0.1 ml may be used instead of vancomycin.)

3. If wound or sclera is involved, consider addition of oral Cipro 250–750 mg BID.

4. Consider obtaining CT scan to rule out intraocular foreign body.

5. If tetanus immunization is not up to date, give tetanus toxoid 0.5 ml IM.

6. Steroids should **Not** be used until fungal organisms are ruled out. If no fungi are isolated, may use prednisolone acetate 1% Q4hr and subconjunctival dexamethasone 4 mg. Prednisone 40–80 mg PO QD is at the discretion of the surgeon. If fungus is isolated, specific antifungal regimens may be used.

7. Incidence of posttraumatic endophthalmitis higher in rural settings; most common agents are *S. epidermidis, Bacillus* species, *Streptococcus* species *S. aureus*, and various fungi.

8. Benefit of subconjunctival antibiotics is limited and is not often used; if used, may consider gentamicin and clindamycin 34 mg, which can be repeated daily.

Endogenous

Notes:

1. Therapy is variable and treatment depends on suspected source.

2. Thorough physical examination must be performed to locate potential source of infection, and consultation with an infectious disease specialist is desirable.

3. Broad-spectrum IV antibiotics are used according to the suspected source of septic infection and blood culture results. IV drug users should receive aminoglycosides and clindamycin to eliminate possible *Bacillus cereus*, and vancomycin should be

Antibacterial Agents

29

considered for *S. aureus* coverage. Other common associated pathogens include *Streptococcus* species and *S. aureus* with endocarditis, and *Candida* with indwelling catheters, hyperalimentation, and IV drug users.

4. Intravitreal antibiotics offer higher intraocular concentrations.
5. Vitrectomy offers the theoretical benefit of reducing infective load and providing sufficient material of diagnostic culture and

pathology.
6. For fungal etiologies (see Subject Index for specific organisms), vitrectomy should be used only if not responsive to systemic medications.

2

Antifungal Agents

AGENTS[1]

Drug	Trade	Preparation	Usual dosage	Notes
amphotericin B[a]	Fungizone	Soln, 0.1–0.5% Subconj Intravitreal IV	Q1–6hr 0.8–1.0 mg 5 μg/0.1 ml 0.8–1.0 mg/kg/day	Varies depending on pathogen
fluconazole[a,b]	Diflucan	PO/IV	400 mg on day 1, then 100–400 mg QD	Max daily dose 400 mg
flucytosine[a]	Ancobon	Soln, 1% PO	Q1–6hr 50–150 mg/kg in 4 divided doses	Varies depending on pathogen Used only as adjunctive treatment; serum levels must be followed
itraconazole[b]	Sporanox	PO	200 mg QD–BID	—
ketoconazole[a,b]	Nizoral	PO	200–400 mg QD	Take with food
miconazole	Monistat	Soln, 1, 2% Subconj Intravitreal	Q1–6hr 5–10 mg 10 μg	Varies depending on pathogen
natamycin	Natacyn	Susp, 5%	Q1–6hr	Varies depending on pathogen

[a]Toxic agent with potential severe side effects—refer to product information and warnings before use. Some side effects are listed below.
[b]Drug has potential to interact with some medications and may precipitate acute ventricular arrythmia (e.g., terfenadine, astemizole, cisapride, triazolam).

[1]Refer to Appendix 3 for activity spectrum of antifungal agents.

SIDE EFFECTS:

Drug	Preparation	Side Effects
amphotericin B[a]	Soln Subconj Intravitreal IV	Burning, irritation Local ischemic necrosis, subconjunctival nodule Cherosis, corneal clouding, poss:ble risk of retinal toxicity We recommend giving in consultation with infectious disease specialist or physician familiar with its use (consider a test dose to monitor for severe reaction). Rapid infusion can result in hypotension, hypokalemia, arrhythmias, and shock. Fever, chills, hypotension, and dyspnea are common. Nephrotoxicity, renal tubular acidosis, electrolyte abnormalities (hypokalemia and hypomagnesemia), anemia, headache, nausea, vomiting, malaise, weight loss, phlebitis, thrombocytopenia, mild leukopenia
fluconazole[a,b]	PO	Gastrointestinal distress, allergic rash, eosinophillia, Stevens–Johnson syndrome, transaminase elevation, thrombocytopenia. Increases concentrations of phenytoin, sulfonylureas, warfarin, and cyclosporine
flucytosine[a]	Soln PO	Burning, irritation (typically less than amphotericin) Marrow suppression leading to leukopenia and thrombocytopenia, rash, nausea, vomiting, severe enterocolitis, hepatotoxicity, renal toxicity, and cardiac arrest
itraconazole[b]	PO	Nausea, vomiting, rash, pruritus, weakness, dizziness, vertigo, pedal edema, paresthesias, impotence, loss of libido
ketoconazole[a,b]	PO	Nausea, anorexia, vomiting, allergic rash, pruritus, gynecomastia, decreased libido/impotence, hypertension, and fluid retention secondary to concentrations of adrenalcortical steroids, elevated liver function tests (LFTs)
miconazole	Soln Subconj	Burning, itching, irritation Generally well tolerated
natamycin	Soln	Less irritating than amphotericin

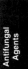

Antifungal
Agents

SPECIFIC ANTIFUNGAL REGIMENS

Special Note on Fungal Keratitis: Although the regimens are given for specific organisms, the major differentiation is between ulcers caused by yeast—for which amphotericin B is the drug of choice—or mold (most commonly *Fusarium*)—for which natamycin is generally the preferred agent. Mechanical debridement of superficial lesions removes necrotic tissue and may aid with antifungal medication penetration. Therapeutic penetrating keratoplasty should be considered for progressive disease or deep penetration to prevent development of endophthalmitis.

Yeast

Candidiasis (*Candida albicans*)

Candida albicans involvement of eye beyond eyelid skin and conjunctivitis is usually part of systemic involvement; therefore, a systemic evaluation is needed.

EYELID SKIN OR CONJUNCTIVAL INVOLVEMENT. Ketoconazole 400 mg PO QD with food.

KERATITIS.[2] Topical amphotericin B drops Q1/2–1hr with either oral ketoconazole, itraconazole, or fluconazole. If no improvement, consider penetrating keratoplasty (PKP). Some advocate addition of flucytosine drops Q1/2–1hr.[3]

RETINITIS/UVEITIS/ENDOPHTHALMITIS.[4] Fluconazole 400 mg PO QD for 3 weeks. In resistant cases, may substitute with intravenous amphotericin B 1 mg/kg/day for total dose of 2 g. Intravitreal amphotericin B 5 μg at time of vitrectomy may also be given. If source is traumatic inoculation, refer to Endophthalmitis in the Subject Index. If source is endogenous, refer to Endophthalmitis— Endogenous in the Subject Index.

Cryptococcus (*Cryptococcus neoformans*)

Must rule out CNS involvement and underlying immunosuppression or AIDS, because meningitis is treated differently.

---

[2] See Special Note on Fungal Keratitis at the beginning of this section.
[3] From *Int Ophthalmol Clin* Summer 1996;36(3):1–15.
[4] Recommend consultation with infectious disease specialist.

KERATITIS.[5] Topical amphotericin B drops Q1/2–1hr with either oral fluconazole, ketoconazole, or itraconazole. If no improvement, consider PKP. Some advocate addition of flucytosine drops Q1/2–1hr.[6]

CHOROIDITIS.[7] If isolated choroiditis, then use amphotericin B 0.5–0.8 mg/kg/day with flucytosine 2 g PO Q6hr for 8 to 10 weeks[8]; weeks if unresponsive or endophthalmitis/significant vitritis develops, may use intravitreal amphotericin B with vitrectomy.[9]

Molds

Aspergillosis (Aspergillus) *(Filamentous Fungus, Septated)*

DACRYOCYSTITIS. Surgical removal of "aspergilloma" with possible surgical reconstruction of nasolacrimal drainage system is the definitive treatment. Antifungal medication is not generally required.

KERATITIS.[10] First choice is topical amphotericin B drops Q1hr initially with oral ketoconazole or fluconazole; second choice of topical agent is natamycin. Consider miconazole drops for infections refractory to amphotericin B and natamycin.

ENDOPHTHALMITIS.[11] Intravitreal and subconjunctival amphotericin B with vitrectomy. Should evaluate for systemic involvement.

ORBITAL INFECTION.[12] Requires surgical debridement with intravenous amphotericin B.

Fusarium *(Filamentous Fungus, Septated)*

KERATITIS.[13] First-choice topical agent is natamycin every 30 min to 1 hr for first 2 days; second-line topical agents are miconazole or flucytosine.

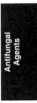

Antifungal Agents

35

[5] See Special Note on Fungal Keratitis at the beginning of this section (see page 34).
[6] From *Int Ophthalmol Clin* Summer 1996;36(3):1–15.
[7] Recommend consultation with infectious disease special.st.
[8] From *Retina* 1990;10:27–32.
[9] From *Retina* 1987;7:75–79.
[10] See Special Note on Fungal Keratitis at the beginning of this section.
[11] Recommend consultation with infectious disease special.st.
[12] Recommend consultation with infectious disease specialist.
[13] See Special Note on Fungal Keratitis at the beginning of this section.

Mucormycosis[14] (Zygomycosis) (*Filamentous Fungus, Nonseptated*)

KERATITIS[15]/ENDOPHTHALMITIS.[16] Due to the highly invasive nature, would recommend local treatment with topical amphotericin B and systemic amphotericin B. Consider surgical debridement.

ORBITAL INFECTION.[17] Use intravenous amphotericin B; may require surgical debridement with topical amphotericin B washings.

Dimorphic Fungi

Blastomycosis[18] (*Blastomyces dermatitidis*)

GRANULOMATOUS BLEPHAROCONJUNCTIVITIS. Itraconazole 200 mg PO QD for 6 months. All extrapulmonary blastomycosis needs to be treated systemically. With severely ill patients, consider systemic amphotericin B.

KERATITIS.[19] As above, with addition of topical miconazole drops.

Coccidioidomycosis[20] (*Coccidioides immitis*)

Note: May get phlyctenular conjunctivitis, episcleritis, or scleritis as part of symptomatic primary infection syndrome "Valley Fever." These are self-limited and do not require treatment, since they are felt to be a hypersensitivity reaction to coccidiodal antigens.

POSTERIOR UVEITIS. Many times, involvement is asymptomatic and resolves spontaneously. Symptomatic involvement (e.g., chronic granulomatous iridocyclitis, choroiditis, and retinitis) is usually associated with progressive systemic coccidiomycosis. Life-threatening disease, such as meningeal involvement, is treated with IV amphotericin B. Non-life-threatening disease may be treated with fluconazole 400 to 600 mg PO QD for 9 to 12 months or itraconazole 200 mg PO BID for 9 to 12 months.

[14] Recommend consultation with infectious disease specialist.
[15] See Special Note on Fungal Keratitis at the beginning of this section.
[16] Recommend consultation with infectious disease specialist.
[17] Recommend consultation with infectious disease specialist.
[18] Recommend consultation with infectious disease specialist.
[19] See Special Note on Fungal Keratitis at the beginning of this section.
[20] Recommend consultation with infectious disease specialist.

Histoplasmosis (*Histoplasma capsulatum*)

CHOROIDITIS. Typically not treated by medications. However, sequelae of choroidal neovascularization must be monitored for potential laser treatment.

Sporotrichosis[21] (*Sporothrix schenckii*)

EYELID SKIN. Ten drops of saturated potassium iodide PO TID; increase until total daily dose of 120 drops. Consider concurrent use of topical amphotericin B. Continue systemic treatment 1 month after skin clears.

GRANULOMATOUS BLEPHAROCONJUNCTIVITIS. Treat as extracutaneous disease; itraconazole 300 mg PO BID for 6 months, then 200 mg PO BID long term.

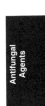

Antifungal
Agents

37

[21] Recommend consultation with infectious disease specialist.

3

Antiviral Agents

TOPICAL

Drug	Trade	Preparation	Usual dosage	Notes[a]
acyclovir	Zovirax	Oint, 3%	5×/day	For HSV keratitis NOT available in U.S.
adenine arabinoside	—	Soln, 1%	Q2hr	For resistant HSV keratitis NOT available in U.S.
idoxuridine	Herplex	Soln, 0.1%	5×/day	For HSV keratitis No longer produced in U.S.
trifluridine	Viroptic	Soln, 1.0%	9×/day; then taper once epithelial defect is healed	Preferred first-line agent for HSV keratitis
			5×/day	For HSV conjunctivitis
vidarabine	Vira-A	Oint, 3.0%	5×/day	For HSV keratitis

[a] HSV, herpes simplex virus.

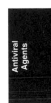

Antiviral
Agents

SYSTEMIC

Note: All have significant side effects which need to be monitored; refer to Side Effects.

Drug	Trade	Dosage	Notes[a]
acyclovir	Zovirax	400 mg PO 5×/day × 7–10 days 800 mg PO 5×/day × 7–10 days	For HSV uveitis/dermatitis For VZV ophthalmicus (if within 72 hr of rash onset)
		5 mg/kg IV Q8hr × 7–10 days	For HSV in immunocompromised patient, adjust dose in renal failure[b]
		10–12 mg/kg IV Q8hr × 7–14 days	For primary/disseminated VZV, adjust dose in renal failure[b]
		1500 mg/m²/day IV in 3 divided doses × 7–10 days	For **acute retinal necrosis**[c] should consider chronic oral suppressive dose; adjust dose in renal failure[b]
cidofovir	Vistide	5 mg/kg IV Q1wk for 2 wk then Q2wk Intravitreal 20 µg Q5–6wk[d]	For CMV retinitis in HIV+ patients; hydration and probenicid[e] must be given with both intravit and IV; adjust dose in renal failure[b]
famciclovir	Famvir	500 mg PO TID × 7 days	For VZV ophthalmicus (if within 72 hr of rash onset)

Antiviral Agents

foscarnet	Foscavir	IV induction 60 mg/kg Q8hr × 2–3 wk IV maintenance 90–120 mg/kg QD × 5–7 days/wk Intravitreal induction 1.2 mg in 0.05 ml 2–3×/wk Intravitreal maintenance 1.2 mg in 0.05 ml Q wk	For CMV retinitis in HIV+ patients; must adjust IV dose in renal failure[b]
		40 mg/kg IVQ8 hr	For HSV infection not responsive to acyclovir
ganciclovir	Cytovene	IV induction 5 mg/kg BID × 2–3 wk IV maintenance 5 mg/kg QD or 6 mg/kg QD 5 days/wk Intravitreal induction 200 µg in 0.1 ml 2–3×/wk for 2–3 wk Intravitreal maintenance 200 µg in 0.1 ml Q1wk Oral maintenance 3 g PO QID	For CMV retinitis in HIV+ patients, must adjust dose in renal failure[b]
	Vitrasert[f]	Sustained release intraocular implant 4.5 mg (1 µg/hr) Continue therapy for 32 wk or until progression of disease despite implant	
valacyclovir	Valtrex	1.0 g PO TID × 7–14 days	For VZV ophthalmicus (within 72 hr of rash onset), 3–5× more bioavailable than acyclovir, not advised in immuno-compromised patients

[a] HSV, herpes simplex virus; VZV, varicella-zoster virus; CMV, cytomegalovirus; HIV, human immunodeficiency virus.

[b] For renal dosing, see Appendix 4.

[c] For acute retinal necrosis, consider addition of systemic steroids and possibly anticoagulation (controversial).

[d] Ten µg intravitreal injection not as effective (Ophthalmology 1997;104:1049–1057).

[e] Probenecid should be given 2 g PO 3 hr prior to cidofovir infusion and 1 g at 2 and 8 hr postinfusion

[f] Arch Ophthalmol 1994;112;1531–1539.

SIDE EFFECTS:

Drug	Preparation	Side Effects
acyclovir	PO	GI disturbances, rash, headache, renal toxicity
	IV	Reversible crystalline nephropathy (avoidable with adequate oral hydration), phlebitis, hallucinations, seizures, coma, encephalopathy
cidofovir	Intravitreal	Iritis, hypotony
	IV	Nephrotoxicity, iritis, hypotony, neutropenia, metabolic acidosis
foscarnet	IV	Nephrotoxicity, Ca and Mg abnormalities, seizures, neutropenia
ganciclovir	IV	Myelosuppression, thrombocytopenia, liver function abnormalities, renal dysfunction, headaches, GI upset, psychiatric disturbances, seizure; do **not** give in conjunction with AZT (worsens neutropenia)
valacyclovir	PO	Possible association with thrombotic thrombocytopenic purpura/hemolytic uremia syndrome in immunocompromised host with high doses, otherwise similar to acyclovir

4

Antiparasitic Agents

PROTOZOA

Acanthamoeba

Note: Give combination of two or three different drops Q1/2–2hr combined with itraconazole 200 mg PO daily.

Drug	Trade	Preparation	Dosage	Notes
propamidine isethionate	Brolene	Soln, 0.1%	Q1/2–2hr	First-line agent
polymyxin B/neomycin/gramicidin	Ak-Spore, Neosporin, Ocuspor-G, Polymycin	Soln, 10,000 U/ 0.35%/0.025%	Q1/2–2hr	First-line agent
polyhexamethylene biguanide	Baquacil	Soln, 0.02%	Q1/2–2hr	First-line agent
chlorhexidine	—	Soln, 0.02%	Q1/2–2hr	Second-line agent
clotrimazole	—	Susp, 1%	Q1–2hr	Second-line agent
dibromopropamidine isethionate	Brolene	Oint, 0.15%	QHS	To be used during taper of Brolene drops

Leishmaniasis

Note: Eyelid lesion can cause conjunctivitis.[1]

Drug	Trade	Dosage
stibogluconate sodium	Pentostam	20 Sb/kg/day IV or IM for 20–28 days
or		
meglumine antimonate	Glucantime	20 Sb/kg/day IV or IM for 20–28 days

Note: Pediatric dosing same for both medications.

Microsporidia (*Encephalitozoon hellem, Nosema corneum*)

Drug	Trade		Notes
fumagillin	Fumidil-B		[a]
or			
itraconazole			[b]

Note: Infections by *E. hellem* have responded to above. No topical regimen exists for *N. corneum* which may need penetrating keratoplasty.

[a] *Am. J Ophthalmol* 1993;115:293.
[b] *Ophthalmology* 1991;98:196.

[1] Regimen from *Med Lett* 1995;37:99–106.

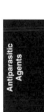

Antiparasitic
Agents

45

Pneumocystis carinii Choroiditis

Drug	Trade	Dosage
trimethoprim/sulfamethoxazole	Bactrim	20 mg/kg IV QD (of TMX component) × 21 days
or		
pentamidine		4 mg/kg IV QD × 21 days

Note: Seen with disseminated disease. Must include systemic evaluation for other sites of disease and immunocompromised status. Pediatric dosing is the same.

Toxoplasmosis Retinochoroiditis (*Toxoplasma gondii*)

Immunosuppressed Patient

Drug	Trade	Dosage for acute infection	Maintenance
pyrimethamine	Daraprim	200 mg PO load, then 50–100 mg PO QD × 3–6 wk	25–50 mg PO QD
plus			
sulfadiazine[a]		1–1.5 g PO or IV Q6hr × 3–6 wk	500 mg–1 g PO Q6hr
plus			
folinic acid[b]		10 mg PO QD × 3–6 wk	10 mg PO QD
clindamycin[c]	—	450–600 mg PO QID or 900 mg IV Q8hr × 3–6 wk	300 mg PO QID

Note: May consider concurrent treatment with oral prednisone (1 mg/kg/day) for inflammation.
[a] If sulfa allergic, may substitute with clindamycin.
[b] Folinic acid is used to avoid pyrimethamine-induced myelosuppression.
[c] If sulfa allergic.

Immunocompetent Patient

Drug	Trade	Dosage
pyrimethamine	Daraprim	100 mg PO, load then 25 mg PO QD for 4–5 wk
plus		
sulfadiazine[a]		1–1.5 mg PO or IV Q6hr for 4–5 wk
plus		
folinic acid[b]		10 mg PO QD for 4–5 wk
clindamycin[c]	—	450 mg PO TID or 900 mg IV Q8hr for 4–5 wk

[a] If sulfa allergic, may substitute with clindamycin.
[b] Folinic acid is used to avoid pyrimethamine-induced myelosuppression.
[c] If sulfa allergic.

Pediatric

Drug	Trade	Dosage
pyrimethamine	Daraprim	2 mg/kg/day × 3 days, then 1 mg/kg/day (max 25 mg/day) × 4 wk
plus		
sulfadiazine[a]		100–200 mg/kg/day × 4 wk
plus		
folinic acid[b]		10 mg PO QD × 4 wk

Note: Congenitally infected newborns should be treated with pyrimethamine and sulfadiazine every 2–3 days for 1 year.
[a] If sulfa allergic, may substitute with clindamycin.
[b] Folinic acid is used to avoid pyrimethamine-induced myelosuppression.

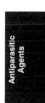

Antiparasitic Agents

Pregnancy

Drug	Trade	Dosage
spiramycin	Rovamycine	3–4 g/day × 3–4 wk

HELMINTHS

Filariasis[2]

Onchocerciasis (Onchocerca volvulus; *"river blindness"*)

Drug	Trade	Dosage
ivermectin	Mectizan 3–12 mo	150 µg/kg single dose, repeated every

Notes: 1. Consider antihistamines or corticosteroids to reduce allergic reaction caused by dead microfilaria.
2. Pediatric dosing is the same.

[2]Regimen from *Med Lett* 1995;37:99–106.

Loasis (Loa loa)

Drug	Trade	Dosage	Notes
diethylcarbamazine	Hetrazan	Day 1: 50 mg PO QD Day 2–3: 50 mg TID Days 4–21:9 mg/kg/day in 3 divided doses	Adult dose
		Day 1: 1 mg/kg PO QD Days 2–3: 1 mg/kg TID Days 4–21: 9 mg/kg/day in 3 divided doses	Pediatric dose

Notes:
1. Heavy filaria burden may induce encephalopathy; may use ivermectin or albendazole or apheresis to reduce microfilarial counts.[3]
2. Consider antihistamines or corticosteroids to reduce allergic reaction caused by dead microfilaria ("Mazzotti reaction").

Tapeworm (*Taenia solium*; "Cysticercosis")

Notes:
1. Antihelminth treatment is usually not indicated for isolated conjunctival or retinal disease, but is indicated for orbital involvement.
2. Consider obtaining computed tomography scan to rule out neurocystercercosis, especially if antihelminth medications are going to be used, since inflammation secondary to death of organism can be fatal.
3. Isolated conjunctival involvement may be treated with surgical excision alone.

[3] From *Infect Dis Clin North Am* 1993;7:619.

Antiparasitic
Agents

4. For posterior segment involvement, laser of worm or vitrectomy to remove organism may be preferable.
5. Antihelminth medical regimens for orbital involvement are not standardized, but some regimens are described. Combination of albendazole or praziquantel in conjunction with prednisone (to decrease inflammation) for 4 weeks has been recommended,[4] although single dose of praziquantel has also been described.[5]

Drug	Trade	Dosage	Notes
albendazole	Zentel	15 mg/kg/day PO × 4 wk	Pediatric dosing same[a]
praziquantel	Biltricide	5–10 mg/kg once	Pediatric dosing same[b]
prednisone	—	1.5–2.0 mg/kg/day × 4 wk	—

[a]*Opthalmology* 1997;104(10):1599–1604.
[b]*Med Lett* 1995;37:99–106.

Toxocariasis (Visceral Larva Migrans; *Toxocara canis*)

Drug	Trade	Dosage	Note
albendazole	Zentel	400 mg PO BID × 3–5 days	Pediatric dosing same

[4]From *Ophtalmology* 1997;104(10):1599–1604.
[5]From *Med Lett* 1995;37:99–106.

5

Antiglaucoma Agents

ALPHA AGONISTS[1] (WHITE TOP—IOPIDINE; PURPLE TOP—ALPHAGAN)

MECHANISM OF ACTION: Activation of alpha-2 receptors in ciliary body inhibits aqueous secretion. Brimonidine also reported to increase uveoscleral outflow.

SIDE EFFECTS: Allergy, mydriasis, dry mouth, dry eye, hypotension, lethargy.

CONTRAINDICATIONS: Monoamine oxidase inhibitor use.

Drug	Trade	Preparation	Usual dosage	Notes
apraclonidine	Iopidine	Soln, 0.5% Soln, 1%	TID Single dose	For short-term use For prophylaxis of postlaser intraocular pressure spike
brimonidine	Alphagan	Soln, 0.2%	TID/BID	Highly selective alpha-2 agonist

BETA BLOCKERS[2] 0.25% LIGHT BLUE TOP, 0.5% YELLOW TOP EXCEPT METIPRANOLOL—WHITE TOP

MECHANISM OF ACTION: Beta blockade in ciliary body reduces intraocular pressure by decreasing aqueous humor production.

SIDE EFFECTS:

Local: Blurred vision, corneal anesthesia, superficial punctate keratopathy.

Systemic: Bradycardia/heart block, bronchospasm, fatigue, impotence, mood change, decreases sensitivity to hypoglycemic symptoms in insulin-dependent diabetics, worsening of myasthenia gravis.

CONTRAINDICATIONS: Asthma, severe chronic obstructive pulmonary disease, bradycardia, heart block, congestive heart failure (CHF), myasthenia gravis.

[1,2]For listing of preservatives of antiglaucoma medications, refer to Appendix 5.

Drug	Trade	Preparation	Usual dosage	Notes
betaxolol	Betoptic-S	Susp, 0.25%	BID	Relatively cardioselective
	Betoptic	Soln, 0.5%	BID	Relatively cardioselective
carteolol	Ocupress	Soln, 1%	BID	Nonselective, has intrinsic sympathomimetic activity
levobunolol	AKBETA, Betagan	Soln, 0.25%, 0.5%	QD–BID	Nonselective (long half-life)
metipranolol	Optipranolol	Soln, 0.3%	BID	Nonselective (White Top)
timolol hemihydrate	Betimol	Soln, 0.25%, 0.5%	BID	Nonselective
timolol maleate	Timoptic	Soln, 0.25%, 0.5%	BID	Nonselective
	Timoptic XE	Soln, 0.25%, 0.5%	QD	Nonselective, gel-forming solution

CARBONIC ANHYDRASE INHIBITORS[3] (ORANGE TOP)

MECHANISM OF ACTION: Inhibition of carbonic anhydrase decreases aqueous production in ciliary body; when given parentally, will also dehydrate the vitreous.

SIDE EFFECTS: Local (with topical therapy): bitter taste.

Systemic with Topical Therapy: diuresis, fatigue, GI upset, Stevens–Johnson syndrome, theoretical risk of aplastic anemia

Systemic with Systemic Therapy: hypokalemic/acidosis, renal stones, paresthesias, nausea, cramps, diarrhea, malaise, lethargy, depression, impotence, unpleasant taste, aplastic anemia, Stevens–Johnson syndrome.

CONTRAINDICATIONS: Sulfa allergy, hyponatremia/kalemia, recent renal stones, thiazide diuretics, digitalis use.

[3]For listing of preservatives of antiglaucoma medications, refer to Appendix 5.

Drug	Trade	Preparation	Usual dosage	Notes
acetazolamide	Diamox	125, 250 mg tabs	QD–QID	Onset within 2 hr, lasts 4–6 hr
	Diamox Sequels	500 mg caps	QD–BID	Lasts 12–24 hr
		500 mg IV	One dose	Immediate onset, duration 4 hr
		5–10 mg/kg/dose	PO TID–QID	For temporary intraocular pressure control in **infantile glaucoma**; definitive treatment is surgical. For preparation instructions see Appendix 2. Also see subject index
dorzolamide	Trusopt	Soln, 2%	BID–TID	TID for single therapy BID when used in combination with beta blockers
methazolamide	Neptazane, MZM, Glauctabs	25, 50 mg tabs	BID–QID	—

HYPEROSMOLAR AGENTS[4]

MECHANISM OF ACTION: Osmotically decreases intraocular fluid volume and intraocular pressure in acute situations.

SIDE EFFECTS:

Mannitol: CHF, urinary retention in men, backache, myocardial infarction, headache, mental confusion.

Glycerin: vomiting, less likely to produce CHF than mannitol, otherwise similar to mannitol.

Isosorbide: same as glycerin, except perhaps safer in diabetes.

CONTRAINDICATIONS: CHF, DKA (glycerin), subdural or subarachnoid hemorrhage, preexisting severe dehydration.

[4]For listing of preservatives of antiglaucoma medications, refer to Appendix 5.

Drug	Trade	Preparation	Usual dosage	Notes
glycerin	Osmoglyn	50% soln	1–1.5 g/kg PO	—
isosorbide	Ismotic	45% soln	1.5 g/kg PO	Onset in 30 min, lasts 5–6 hr
mannitol	Osmitrol	5%–20% soln	0.5–2 g/kg IV	Onset 30–60 min, lasts 6 hr; infuse over 45 min

MIOTICS[5] (GREEN TOP)

MECHANISM OF ACTION: Direct cholinergics stimulate muscarinic receptors, indirect cholinergics block acetylcholinesterase: Miotics cause pupillary muscle constriction, which is believed to pull open the trabecular meshwork to increase trabecular outflow.

SIDE EFFECTS:

Direct Cholinergic.

   Local: brow ache, breakdown of blood/aqueous barrier, angle closure (increases pupillary block and causes the lens/iris diaphragm to move anteriorly), decreased night vision, variable myopia, retinal tear/detachment, and possibly anterior subcapsular cataracts.

   Systemic: rare.

Indirect Cholinergic

   Local: retinal detachment, cataract, myopia, intense miosis, angle closure, increased bleeding postsurgery, punctal stenosis, increased formation of posterior synechiae in chronic uveitis.

   Systemic: diarrhea, abdominal cramps, enuresis, increases effect of succinylcholine.

CONTRAINDICATIONS:

Direct Cholinergic: peripheral retinal pathology, central media opacity, young patient (increases myopic effect), uveitis.

Indirect Cholinergic: succinylcholine administration, predisposition to retinal tear, anterior subcapsular cataract, ocular surgery, uveitis.

[5]For listing of preservatives of antiglaucoma medications, refer to Appendix 5.

Antiglaucoma Agents

Drug	Trade	Preparation	Usual dosage	Notes
echothiophate iodide	Phospholine Iodide	Soln, 0.03%, 0.06%, 0.125%, 0.25%	QD–BID	Indirect, avoid in phakic patients
physostigmine	Isopto Eserine	Soln, 0.25%, 0.5%	QD–BID	Indirect, avoid in phakic patients
	Eserine	Oint, 0.25%	Unit dose	Indirect, used postoperatively
demecarium bromide	Humorsol	Soln, 0.125%, 0.25%	QD–BID	Indirect
acetylcholine	Miochol-E	1:100 dilution	Inject into anterior chamber	Direct, used during surgery
carbachol	Isopto Carbachol	Soln, 0.75%, 1.5%, 2.25%, 3%	QD–TID	Direct/indirect
	Carbastat, Miostat	Soln, 0.01%	Inject into anterior chamber	Direct/indirect, used during surgery
pilocarpine hydrochloride	Isopto Carpine, Pilocar, Piloptic	Soln, 0.25%–8%	QID	Direct
	Akarpine, Pilostat, Storzine	Soln, 0.5%, 1%, 2%, 3%, 4%, 6%	QID	Direct
		Soln, 1%, 2%, 4%	QID	Direct
	Pilopine HS gel	Oint, 4%	QHS	Direct
	Ocusert Pilo 20	Insert, 20 µg	Q wk	Direct
	Ocusert Pilo 40	Insert, 40 µg	Q wk	Direct
pilocarpine nitrate	Pilagan	Soln, 1%, 2%, 4%	QID	Direct

PROSTAGLANDINS[6] (CLEAR TOP)

MECHANISM OF ACTION: Prostaglandin PF agonist, which increases uveoscleral outflow.

SIDE EFFECTS:

Local: increase in melanin pigmentation in iris, blurred vision, eyelid redness; cystoid macular edema and anterior uveitis has been reported.

Systemic: systemic upper respiratory infection symptoms, backache, chest pain, myalgia.

CONTRAINDICATIONS: pregnancy, consider not using in inflammatory conditions.

Drug	Trade	Preparation	Usual dosage
latanaprost	Xalatan	Susp, 0.005%	QHS

Note: Must be refrigerated prior to opening; good for 6 weeks once open.

Antiglaucoma Agents

[6]For listing of preservatives of antiglaucoma medications, refer to Appendix 5.

SYMPATHOMIMETIC[7] (PURPLE TOP)

MECHANISM OF ACTION: In ciliary body, the response is variable (beta stimulation increases aqueous production, but alpha stimulation decreases aqueous production); in trabecular meshwork, beta stimulation causes increased trabecular outflow and increased uveoscleral outflow; overall effect lowers intraocular pressure.

SIDE EFFECTS:

Local: cystoid macular edema in aphakia, mydriasis, rebound hyperemia, blurred vision, adenochrome deposits, allergic blepharoconjunctivitis.

Systemic: tachycardia/ectopy, hypertension, headache.

CONTRAINDICATIONS: narrow angles, aphakia, pseudophakia, soft lenses, hypertension, cardiac disease.

Drug	Trade	Preparation	Usual dosage	Notes
dipivefrin	Propine	Soln, 0.1%	BID	Prodrug of epinephrine
epinephrine	Epifrin, Glaucon	Soln, 0.5%, 1%, 2%	BID	Mixed alpha and beta agonist

[7]For listing of preservatives of antiglaucoma medications, refer to Appendix 5.

COMBINATION AGENT[8]

Drug	Trade	Preparation	Usual dosage	Note
epinephrine/pilocarpine	E-Pilo	Soln, 1%/1%, 2%, 4%, 6%	QID	Miotic with sympathomimetic agent

SPECIFIC REGIMENS

Infantile/Congenital Glaucoma

Notes:
1. Definitive treatment is surgical (e.g., goniotomy, trabeculotomy, trabeculectomy, tube shunt, etc.), which should be performed as soon as possible.
2. Medical treatment is done only temporarily until appropriate surgery can be performed or to clear the cornea to aid in surgical management.
3. For initial medical treatment, we use oral acetazolamide 5 to 10 mg/kg/dose TID–QID (for preparation instructions, see Appendix 2). This may be supplemented with timolol alone[9] or with timolol and pilocarpine 2%.[10]
4. Consultation with an ophthalmologist specializing in either pediatrics or glaucoma is recommended.

[8] For listing of preservatives of antiglaucoma medications, refer to Appendix 5.
[9] From Hoskins HD, Kass MA. *Becker-Shaffer's Diagnosis and therapy of the glaucomas*, 6th ed. St. Louis: Mosby–Year Book, 1989:605–623.
[10] From *Acta Ophthalmol Scand* 1995;73:261–263.

Antiglaucoma Agents

Acute Angle-Closure Glaucoma

Notes: 1. Regimen outlined below is once acute-angle-closure glaucoma secondary to pupillary block has been established. Refer to *Wills Eye Manual*[11] for discussion on evaluation to rule out other etiologies (plateau iris, neovascular glaucoma, uveitic, malignant glaucoma (ciliary block), Posner–Schlossman syndrome, etc.).

2. Definitive treatment is surgical (laser iridectomy, surgical iridectomy, etc.).

3. Medical treatment is needed to facilitate surgical management.

4. Unless contraindicated, we use topical agents (beta blockers, alpha agonists, and carbonic anhydrase inhibitors), systemic carbonic anhydrase inhibitors (do not use sustained-release Diamox Sequels), hyperosmolar agents, and topical steroids.

[11]From Cullom RD, Chang B, eds. *The Wills eye manual: office and emergency room diagnosis and treatment of eye disease*, 2nd ed. Philadelphia: JB Lippincott Co, 1994.

6

Neuro-ophthalmology

AGENTS USED IN NEURO-OPHTHALMOLOGY

Drug	Trade	Preparation	Usual dosage	Notes
botulinum toxin	Botox	Injection	Varies depending on the entity being treated	Used in treatment of blepharospasm, strabismus, and hemifacial spasm
cocaine	N/A[a]	Soln, 10%	1 drop, repeat in 1 min	Used in diagnosis of Horner's syndrome[b]
edrophonium chloride	Tensilon	IV Soln, 10 mg/ml	2–3 mg IV (0.2–0.3 cc)[c]	Used in diagnosis of myasthenia gravis[b]; if unresponsive and no side effects seen after 1 min, may give 0.4 cc Q30sec × 2
hydroxyamphetamine	Paredrine	Soln, 1%	1 drop, repeat in 1 min	Used in diagnosis of Horner's syndrome[b]
methylprednisolone sodium	Solu-Medrol	IV Soln	250 mg IV Q6hr	Treatment of optic neuritis and giant cell arteritis (see below for further discussion)
			Special (see below)	Traumatic optic neuropathy
pilocarpine	N/A	Soln, 0.125%	1 drop	Lower strength used in diagnosis and treatment of Adie's pupil[b]

[a] N/A, not available.
[b] For protocol, refer to Cullom RD, Chang B, eds. *The Wills eye manual: office and emergency room diagnosis and treatment of eye disease*, 2nd ed. Philadelphia: JB Lippincott Co, 1994.
[c] Potential for causing cholinergic crisis, treatment of which includes IV atropine.

SPECIFIC REGIMENS

Giant Cell Arteritis[1]

Notes: 1. Opinions on treatment vary among rheumatologists and among neuro-ophthalmologists. Some feel oral prednisone 10 mg BID is sufficient[2]. Others have written that if **no** visual symptoms have occurred, oral prednisone 60 to 80 mg per day is adequate.[3]

2. Most patients seen at Wills have visual symptoms and we recommend high-dose intravenous methylprednisolone.[4]

Drug	Trade	Preparation	Dosage
methylprednisolone sodium	Solu-Medrol	IV Soln	250 mg IV Q6hr × 3 days Day 4: begin taper with oral prednisone

Optic Neuritis[5]

Notes: 1. Intravenous steroids may speed the recovery of visual acuity.
2. Oral steroids do not hasten recovery time of visual acuity and may worsen the relapse rate.

[1] Consultation with neuro-ophthalmologist is recommended c̄or duration of taper.
[2] From *J Rheumatol* 1990;17:1340–1345.
[3] From *Ann Intern Med* 1978;188:162–167, *Surv Ophthalmoi* 1976;20:547–560, and *Am Heart J* 1980;100:99–107, as discussed in *Arch Fam Med* 1994;3:623–627.
[4] From *Arch Farm Med* 1994;3:623–627.
[5] Consultation with neuro-ophthalmologist is recommended c̄or duration of taper.

Neuroophthalmology

Drug	Trade	Preparation	Dosage	Note
methylprednisolone sodium	Solu-Medrol	IV Soln	250 mg IV Q6hr × 3 days Day 4: begin taper	[a]

[a] *N Engl J Med* 1993;329:1764–1769.

Traumatic Optic Neuropathy[6]

Note: This is an experimental alternative protocol to decompressive surgery; definitive treatment has not been established.[7]

Drug	Trade	Preparation	Dosage
methylprednisolone sodium	Solu-Medrol	IV Soln	30 mg/kg IV load (2 g for healthy adult), then **either** 4.0 mg/kg/hr continuous IV infusion × 24 hr **or** additional 15 mg/kg 2 hr later and 15 mg/kg (1 g in healthy adults) Q6hr × 72 hr

[6] Consultation with neuro-ophthalmologist is recommended for duration of taper.
[7] From *Sem Ophthalmol* 1994;9(3):200–211.

7

Antiinflammatory Agents

STEROIDAL

Notes: 1.   Suspensions are more lipophilic and penetrate the cornea more easily than solutions.
2.   Relative antiinflammatory potency as follows.

Intravenous or intravitreal	Relative Potency	Topical	
cortisone	0.8	Low potency:	Cortisone
cortisol (endogenous)	1		Hydrocortisone
hydrocortisone (synthetic)	1	Mild potency:	Fluorometholone
prednisone	4		Medrysone
prednisolone	4	Moderate potency:	Fluoromethalone acetate
methylprednisolone	5		Dexamethasone phosphate
triamcinolone	5		Prednisolone phosphate
betamethasone	25	High potency:	Rimexolone
dexamethasone	25		Dexamethasone acetate
fluoromethalone	40–50	Highest potency:	Prednisolone acetate

Topical

Drug	Trade	Preparation	Usual dosage
		Used primarily for dermatologic/ rheumatologic conditions	
cortisone	Cortone		
dexamethasone acetate	AK-Dex, Decadron	Susp, 0.1%	Variable
	AK-Dex, Decadron	Oint, 0.05%	Variable
dexamethasone phosphate	Decadron, AK-Dex	Soln, 0.1%	Variable
flucromethalone	Fluro-op, FML	Susp, 0.1%	QOD–QID
	FML Forte	Susp, 0.25%	QOD–QID
	FML S.O.P.	Oint, 0.1%	QD–QID
fluoromethalone acetate	Eflone. Flarex	Susp, 0.1%	QOD–QID
hydrocortisone	Exists only in combination with antibiotic.		
medrysone	HMS Liquifilm	Susp, 1%	QD–Q4hr
prednisolone acetate	Pred Mild	Susp, 0.12%	Variable
	Econopred	Susp, 0.125%	Variable
	Pred Forte, Econopred Plus	Susp, 1%	Variable
prednisolone phosphate	AK-Pred, Inflamase Mild, Pred-Phosphate	Soln, 0.125%	Variable
	AK-Pred, Inflamase Forte, Pred-Phosphate	Soln, 1%	Variable
rimexolone	Vexol	Susp, 1%	Variable

Antiinflammatory Agents

67

Subtenons/Systemic

Drug	Trade	Preparation	Usual dosage	Notes[a]
triamcinolone	Kenalog	Susp, 40 mg/ml	0.5–1.0 ml	Subtenons for uveitis and CME; lasts weeks to months
betamethasone sodium/acetate	Celestone (Soluspan)	Susp, 6 mg/ml	0.5–1.0 ml	Subtenons after ocular surgery, uveitis, and CME; last days to weeks
dexamethasone sodium	Decadron	Soln, 4 mg/ml	0.4 mg in 0.1 ml	Intravitreal injection for endophthalmitis
methylprednisolone acetate	Depo-Medrol	Susp, 80 mg/ml	0.5–1.0 ml	Subtenons for uveitis and CME; lasts months; do not use in patients with steroid responsive glaucoma
methylprednisolone sodium	Solu-Medrol	IV Soln	See Subject Index for further discussion of giant cell arteritis, optic neuritis, and traumatic optic neuropathy	
prednisone	—	1, 2.5, 5, 10, 20, 50 mg tabs	Variable	

[a]CME, Cystoid Macular Edema.

COMBINATION STEROID WITH ANTIBIOTIC

Drug	Trade	Preparation[b]	Usual dosage	Notes[a]
dexamethasone acetate/neomycin/ polymyxin B	Maxitrol, Neopolydex, Ocu-trol, W-DNP	Susp, 0.1%	QD–QID	BC antibiotic with high-potency steroid
dexamethasone (as salt)/tobramycin	Tobradex	Oint, 0.1%	QD–QID	BC antibiotic with high-potency steroid
dexamethasone acetate/tobramycin	Tobradex	Susp, 0.1%	QD–QID	BC antibiotic with high-potency steroid
dexamethasone (as salt)/neomycin	Dexacidin	Oint, 0.1%	QD–QID	BC antibiotic with high-potency steroid
dexamethasone phosphate/neomycin	Dexacidin, Necdecadron, Necdexasone	Soln, 0.1%	QD–Q1hr	BC antibiotic with moderate-potency steroid
fluorometholone/sulfacetamide	Neodecadron FML-S	Oint, 0.5% Susp. 0.1%/10%	QD–QID QD–QID	BS antibiotic with mild-potency steroid
hydocortisone/neomycin/polymyxin B	Cortimycin, Cortisporin	Susp, 1%	QD–QID	BC antibiotic with low-potency steroid
	Cortimycin, Cortisporin	Oint	QD–QID	BC antibiotic with low-potency steroid
hydrocortisone/neomycin/polymyxin B/gramicidin	AK-Spore H.C.	Susp, 1%	QD–QID	BC antibiotic with low-potency steroid

continued

Antiinflammatory Agents

Drug	Trade	Preparation	Usual dosage	Notes[a]
hydrocortisone/oxytetracycline/ polymyxin B	AK-Spore H.C. Terra-Cortril	Oint Susp, 1.5%/ 0.5%/10,000 U	QD–QID TID	BC antibiotic with low-potency steroid
prednisolone acetate/gentamicin	Pred-G	Susp, 0.1%/0.3%	QD–QID	BC antibiotic with high-potency steroid
prednisolone acetate/neomycin/ polymyxin B	Pred-G S.O.P. Poly-Pred	Oint, 0.1%/0.3% Susp, 0.5%	QD–QID QD–QID	BC antibiotic with high-potency steroid
prednisolone acetate/sulfacetamide	AK-Cide	Susp, 0.1%/10%	QD–QID	BS antibiotic with high-potency steroid
prednisolone acetate/sulfacetamide	Blephamide	Susp, 0.2%/10%	QD–QID	BS antibiotic with high-potency steroid
prednisolone acetate/sulfacetamide	Blephamide Cetapred	Oint, 0.2%/10% Susp, 0.25%/10%	QD–QID QD–QID	BS antibiotic with high-potency steroid
prednisolone acetate/sulfacetamide	Metimyd	Susp, 0.5%/10%	QD–QID	BS antibiotic with high-potency steroid
prednisolone acetate/sulfacetamide	Metimyd Sulster, Vasocidin	Oint, 0.5%/10% Soln, 0.23%/10%	QD–QID QD–QID	BS antibiotic with high-potency steroid
prednisolone phosphate/sulfacetamide	Vasocidin	Oint, 0.5%/10%	QD–QID	BS antibiotic with moderate-potency steroid

[a]BC, bacteriocidal; BS, bacteriostatic.
[b]Only strength of steriod is listed for most entries.

NONSTEROIDAL

Note: *Relative contraindication*—triad asthma (asthma in combination with asprin sensitivity and nasal polyposis).

Drug	Trade	Preparation	Usual dosage	Notes
diclofenac	Voltaren	Soln, 0.1%	QID	Indicated for post-cataract-surgery inflammation and treatment of photophobia after incision refractive surgery
flurbiprofen	Ocufen	Soln, 0.03%	2 drops @ 3, 2, 1 hrs. before surgery	Indicated for intraoperative miosis inhibition
ketorolac	Acular	Soln, 0.5%	QID	Indicated for ocular itching and pain and treatment of post-cataract-surgery inflammation
suprofen	Profenal	Soln, 1%	1 drop Q30 min starting 2 hr before surgery	Indicated for intraoperative miosis inhibition

Antiinflammatory Agents

71

8

Mydriatics, Cycloplegics, and Reversal Agents

Drug	Trade	Concentration	Usual dosage/indication	Notes
atropine	Atropisol, Isopto Atropine, Ocu-tropine Ocu-tropine	Soln, 0.5%, 1%, 2%, 3% Oint, 1%	BID–TID (hyphema/ inflammation) BID–3×/wk (inflammation/ pediatric refraction)	Anticholinergic agent[a] Duration 7–14 days Useful in infants/children
cyclopentolate	AK-Pentolate, Cyclogel Ocu-pentolate, Pentolair	Soln, 0.5%, 1%, 2% Soln, 1%	TID–QID (inflammation)	Anticholinergic agent[a] Increased risk of CNS toxicity (psychotic rxn) in children Duration 1–2 days
dapiprazole	Rev-Eyes	Soln, 0.5%	1 drop (reverse dilation)	Alpha blocker, reverses mydriasis from phenylephrine and to lesser extent tropicamide
homatropine	Isopto Homatropine	Soln, 2%, 5%	BID–TID (inflammation)	Anticholinergic agent[a] Duration 3 days; better for children

continued

Drug	Trade	Concentration	Usual dosage/indication	Notes
phenylephrine	AK-Dilate, Mydfrin, Neo-Synephrine, Ocu-phrin AK-Nefrin, Ocu-phrin	Soln, 2.5%, 10% Soln, 0.12%	1 drop (mydriasis)	Adrenergic agent Duration 3–5 hr
scopolamine	Isopto Hyoscine	Soln, 0.25%	BID–TID (inflammation)	Anticholinergic agent[a] Duration 3–7 days; better for children
tropicamide	Mydriacyl, Ocu-tropic, Topicacyl	Soln, 0.5%, 1%	1 drop (cycloplegia)	Anticholinergic agent[a] Duration 4-6 hr
tropicamide/ hydroxy- amphetamine hydrobromide	Paremyd	Soln, 1%/0.25%	1 drop (mydriasis)	Anticholinergic agent[a] with adrenergic agent
scopolamine/ phenylephrine	Murocoll 2	Soln, 0.3%/10%	1 drop (mydriasis)	Anticholinergic agent[a] with adrenergic agent

[a] Anticholineric agents are cycloplegics.

9

Lubricants and Viscoelastics

ARTIFICIAL TEARS, VISCOELASTICS, AND LUBRICATING OINTMENTS

Notes:
1. Viscosity of water is 0.7 centistokes.[1]
2. centistokes (cs) × density = centipoits (cp).
3. centipoits·seconds = cps.
4. *Boric acid* is a balanced salt solution used to equalize osmolarity.

Low Viscosity

Low-viscosity lubricants are useful in mildly symptomatic **dry eyes;** they have a low tendency to blur vision, but typically their effects do not last very long.

Trade name	Viscosity	Osmolarity[a]	Preservative
Preservative free			
Bion Tears	5–15 cps[b]/4.5 cs[c]	270–330	N
Cellufresh	3.2 cp[d]	270–340	N
Dry Therapy	0.7 cs[c]	N/A	N
Refresh	5 cp[d]/2.8 cs[c]	250–305	N
Refresh Plus	3 cp[d]/2.0 cs[c]	270–340	N
Tears Naturale Free	5–15 cp[b]/4.3 cs[c]	270–330	N
Preserved			
AKWA Tears	3.5 cp	250–310	2, 3
GenTeal	7 cps[e]/3.6 cs[c]	220	7
Hypotears	<5 cps[e]/1.2 cs[c]/2.8 cp[d]	220	2, 3
Hypotears PF	<5 cps[e]/1.2 cs[c]/2.8 cp[d]	220	2
Isopto Plain	15–30 cps[b]	270–330	3

Isopto Tears	15–30 cps[b]	270–330	3
Liquifilm Tears	4 cp[d]	220–270	4
Murine	2.3 cp[f]	260	2, 3
Puralube Tears	5 cp[g]	N/A	2, 3
Refresh Tears	3.0 cp[d]	280	1
Tearisol	10–30 cp[e]	220	2, 3
Tears Naturale	5–15 cp[b]/3.7 cs[c]/7.0 cp[d]	270–330	3
Tears Naturale II	6–12 cp[b]/4.0 cs[c]	270–330	5
Tears Plus	4 cp[d]/2.8 cs[c]	260–310	4

N, None; 1, Purite; 2, EDTA; 3, benzalkonium chloride; 4, chlorobutanol; 5, polyquad; 6, sorbic acid; 7, sodium perborate; 8, methyl propylparbens.

[a] N/A, not available;

[b] 25 C, measured on Brookfield Digital Cone and Plate Viscometer (provided by Alcon file data).

[c] 37 C, measured on Cannon–Fenske Viscometer (provided by Stortz advertisement).

[d] 25 C, shear rate 2.6/sec (provided by Allergan file data).

[e] Measured on Brookfield Digital Cone and Plate Viscometer (provided by CIBA file data).

[f] 25 C, measured on Brookfield Digital Cone and Plate Viscometer (provided by Ross file data).

[g] 25 C, measured on Brookfield Digital Cone and Plate Viscometer (provided by Fougera file data).

High Viscosity

High-viscosity lubricants are useful in severely symptomatic **dry eyes;** they have a tendency to blur vision, but last longer than low-viscosity products. If symptoms are not controlled by artifical tears, consider temporary or permanent punctal occlusion therapy; tarsorraphy may be considered for severe cases of exposure keratopathy.

[1] At 37 C, measured on a Cannon–Fenske Viscometer (provided by Stortz advertisement).

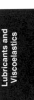

Lubricants and
Viscoelastics

Trade name	Viscosity	Osmolarity	Preservative
Preservative free			
Aquasite PF	250–750 cps[a]/ 800 cp[b]	235	N
Celluvisc	170 cs[c]/ 200–300 cp[b]	270–350	N
Ocucoat PF	46 cs[c]	285 + 32	N
Preserved			
Aquasite	250–750 cps[a]/ 800 cp[b]	235	2
Ocucoat	46 cs[c]	285 + 32	3
Ultra Tears	100–300 cps[d]	270–330	3

[a]Measured on a Brookfield Digital Cone and Plate Viscometer (provided by CIBA file data).
[b]25 C, shear rate 2.6/sec (provided by Allergan file data).
[c]37 C, measured on a Cannon–Fenske Viscometer (provided by Stortz advertisement).
[d]25 C, measured on a Brookfield Digital Cone and Plate Viscometer (provided by Alcon file data).

Unknown Viscosity

Trade name	Viscosity	Osmolarity	Preservative
Comfort Tears	N/A[a]	N/A	2, 3
Dry Eyes	N/A	N/A	3
Murocel	N/A	N/A	8
Theratears	N/A	170	N

[a]N/A, not available.

Viscoelastics

Trade name	Viscosity
Amvisc	62,000 cp[a]
Amvisc Plus	82,000 cp[a]
Healon	200,000 cp[a]
HealonGV	2,000,000 cp[a]
IVISC	140,000 mPa.s[b]
IVISC+	430,000 mPa.s[b]
Ocucoat	4,000 cp[c]
Optimize Viscoelastic	50,000 cp[c]
Provisc	135,000 cp[a]
Viscoat	50,000 cp[a]
Visilon	4,100 cp[c]
Vitrax	35,000 cp[a]

[a]37 C, shear rate 0/sec (provided by Pharmacia advertisement).
[b]Provided by Allergan file data.
[c]Shear rate 2/sec (provided by Mentor file data).
[d]Provided by Shah & Shah IOL Ltd.

Ointments

Lanolin-containing (trade name)	Lanolin-free (trade name)
AKWA TearsOintment	Duolube
Dry Eyes Lubricant	Hypo Tears
Dry Eyes Ointment	Peralube
Duratears Naturale	
Lacri-Lube S.O.P	
LubriTears	
Refresh P.M.	

IRRIGATING SOLUTIONS

Trade name	Preservative[a]
AK-Rinse	2
Blinx	3
Collyrium	1
Dacriose	2
Eye Stream	2
Irrigate	2
Lavoptik Eye Wash	2
M/Rinse	1

[a] 1, Thimerosal; 2, benzalkonium chloride; 3, phenylmercuric acetate.

10

Miscellaneous Agents

AGENTS FOR RELIEF OF SEASONAL ALLERGIC CONJUNCTIVITIS/OCULAR DISCOMFORT

Drug	Trade	Preparation	Usual dosage	Notes
cromolyn sodium	Crolom	Soln, 4%	QID–Q4hr	Mast cell stabilizer; may take weeks for effect
levocabastine	Livostin	Soln, 0.05%	BID–QID	H1 antagonist (preservative may damage contact lenses)
lodoxamide	Alomide	Soln, 0.1%	QID × 2–3 wk	Mast cell inhibitor, possibly faster onset than cromolyn
olopatadine	Patanol	Soln, 0.1%	BID	H1 antagonist with mast cell stabilization

OCULAR DECONGESTANTS

Drug	Trade	Preparation	Usual dosage	Notes
naphazoline	Allergy Drops, Digest 2, Naphcon	Soln, 0.012%	QID PRN	Alpha agonist
	Comfort Eye Drops	Soln, 0.03%	QID PRN	
	AK-Con, Napha-Forte, Naphcon Forte, Nafazair, Vasocon	Soln, 0.1%	QID PRN	
	Opcon Maximum Strength, Allergy Drops	Soln, 0.3%	QID PRN	
naphazoline/glycerin	Clear Eyes	Soln, 0.012%/0.2%	QID PRN	Alpha agonist/artificial tear

naphazoline/polyvinyl alcohol	Albalon VasoClear	Soln, 0.1%/1.4% Soln, 0.02%/2.5%	QID PRN	Alpha agonist/artificial tear
naphazoline/polyvinyl alcohol/zinc sulfate	VasoClear A	Soln, 0.02%/2.5%	QID PRN	Alpha agonist/artificial tear/ astringent[a]
naphazoline/glycerin/zinc sulfate	Clear Eyes ACR	Soln, 0.012%/0.2%/0.25%	QID PRN	alpha agonist/artificial tear/ astringent[a]
naphazoline/pheiramine	Naphcon-A, Napha-A, OcuHist	Soln, 0.025%/0.3%	QID PRN	Alpha agonist/antihistamine
naphazoline/antazoline	Vasocon-A	Soln, 0.05%/0.5%	QID PRN	Alpha agonist/antihistamine
oxymetazoline	Ocuclear, Visine L.R.	Soln, 0.025%	QID PRN	Alpha agonist
phenylephrine	AK-Nefrin, Ocu-Phrin	Soln, 0.12%	QID PRN	Alpha agonist
phenylephrine/ zinc sulfate	Zinefrin	Soln, 0.12%/0.25%	QID PRN	Alpha agonist/astringent[a]
tetrahydrozoline	Eye Drops Regular, Eyesine, Murine Flus, Visine	Soln, 0.05%	QID PRN	Alpha agonist
tetrahydrozoline/ zinc sulfate	Eye Drops AC, Visine AC	Soln, 0.05%/0.25%	QID PRN	Alpha agonist/astringent[a]
tetrahydrozoline/ polyethylene glycol	Visine Moisturizing Drops	Soln, 0.05%	QID PRN	Alpha agonist/artificial tear

[a] Astringents help clear mucus by precipitating proteins.

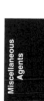

Miscellaneous
Agents

TOPICAL HYPEROSMOLAR AGENTS

Drug	Trade	Preparation	Usual dosage	Notes
glycerin	Ophthalgen	—	1 drop prior to exam	Diagnostic agent used to clear edematous cornea
sodium chloride	Muro-128	Soln, 2%, 5%	QD–Q3hr	Therapeutic agent to dehydrate the cornea
	AK-NaCl, NaCl 5%	Soln, 5%	QD–Q3hr	
	AK-NaCl, Muro-128, NaCl	Oint, 5%	QD–Q3hr	
glucose	Glucose 40 Ophthalmic	Oint, 40%	—	Therapeutic agent

VITAMINS

Drug	Trade	Preparation	Dosage	Notes
N/A[a]	I-Caps	Tablets	1 tab PO QD	Zinc and antioxidant vitamin supplement with more vitamin E and vitamin A than I-Caps Plus
N/A	I-Caps Plus	Tablets	1 tab PO QD	Zinc and antioxidant vitamin supplement plus manganese
N/A	I-Sense	Tablets	1 tab PO QD	Zinc and antioxidant vitamin supplement
N/A	Ocuvite	Tablets	1 tab PO QD	Zinc and antioxidant vitamin supplement
N/A	Ocuvite Extra	Tablets	1 tab PO QD	Zinc and antioxidant vitamin supplement with vitamin B, all in higher concentration than Ocuvite
N/A	Viva-Drops	Soln	1 drop PRN	Lubricant with antioxidants

ANESTHETIC AGENTS
Topical Anesthetics[1]

Drug	Trade	Preparation	Dosage	Notes
cocaine hydrochloride	N/A[a]	Soln, 1%–4%	1 drop	Duration 20–45 min, pupillary dilation, potentiates epinephrine
proparacaine	AK-Taine, Alcaine, Ophthaine, Ophthetic	Soln, 0.5%	1 drop	Duration 15–30 min. Ester linkage
tetracaine	AK-T-Caine, Pontocaine	Soln, 0.5%	1 drop	Duration 9–24 min Ester linkage

[a]N/A, not available.
Note: Topical anesthetics should **only** be used to allow the clinician to perform ocular procedures. They are **not** indicated for use by the patient and should **never** be prescribed.

[1]From Stewart WB, ed. *Surgery of the eyelid, orbit, and lacrimal system*, Monograph 8. San Francisco: American Academy of Ophthalmology, 1993.

Miscellaneous Agents

85

Local Anesthetics[2]

To convert percent solutions to mg/ml, multiply by 10; e.g., 1% = 10 mg/ml.

Drug	Trade	Preparation	Maximum adult dose	Duration of action	Pain on injection[a]	Linkage[b]
bupivacaine	Marcaine	Soln, 0.25%–0.75%	23 ml of 0.75% soln	3–12 hr	5	Amide
lidocaine	Xylocaine					Amide
	w/oepinephrine	Soln, 1%–2%	15 ml of 2% soln	60–75 min	1	
	w/epinephrine	Soln, 1%–2%	25 ml of 2% soln	2 hr	2	
mepivacaine	Carbocaine	Soln, 1%–2%	15 ml of 2% soln	2–3 hr	4	Amide
procaine	Novocain	Soln, 1%–4%	38 ml of 2% soln	30–45 min	3	Ester

[a] 1, least painful; 5, most painful.
[b] Allergic cross-reactions between groups do not occur. If patient is allergic to ester compounds, amides may be tried.

[2] From Stewart WB, ed. *Surgery of the eyelid, orbit, and lacrimal system*, Monograph 8. San Francisco: American Academy of Ophthalmology, 1993.

Adjuncts[3]

Drug	Trade	Preparation	Usual dosage	Notes
hyaluronidase	Wydase	Lyophilized, 150 U/vial	1 vial in 10 ml anesthetic	Depolymerizes polysaccharides and increases effective area of anesthesia, decreases duration of local anesthesia
lidocaine	Xylocaine	1%, nonpreserved, without epinephrine	0.5 ml	**Intraocular** adjunct for cataract surgery, do with "topical anesthesia"
sodium bicarbonate	—	1 mEq/ml	1 ml in 10 ml anesthetic	Decreases pain on injection

MISCELLANEOUS

Drug	Trade	Preparation	Usual dosage	Notes
acetylcysteine	Mucomyst	Soln, 10%, 20% intraocular	QID	For **filamentary keratopathy**
alteplase	Activase		3–6 μg	For clot dissolution postvitrectomy
aminocaproic acid	Amicar	Syrup, 250 mg/ml Tabs, 500 mg	50 mg/kg PO Q4hr (max dose 30 g/day)	For **hyphema**[a,b] Orthostatic hypotension is significant side effect
disodium EDTA	Endrate	Soln, 15%	Applied by physician	For **band keratopathy**[b] Do **not** use dicalcium EDTA

[3]From Stewart WB, ed. *Surgery of the eyelid, orbit, and lacrimal system*, Monograph 8. San Francisco: American Academy of Ophthalmology, 1993.

continued

Miscellaneous Agents

Drug	Trade	Preparation	Usual dosage	Notes
cyclosporine	—	Soln, 2% (in oil)	QID	For **ligneous conjunctivitis** and other inflammatory conditions
cysteamine	—	Soln, 0.5%	Q1hr while awake	For **cystinosis** corneal crystals[c]
hydroxypropyl cellulose	Lacrisert	Insert, 5 mg	QD–BID	For moderate to severe dry eye syndrome
silver nitrate	—	Soln, 1% (in wax ampules)	Applied by physician	For **superior limbic keratoconjuntivitis**[b]; do **not** use sticks or higher concentration solutions
tyloxapol	Enuclene	Soln, 0.25%	TID–QID PRN	Cleaning/lubricating solution for artificial eyes
white petrolatum/ mineral oil/steric acid	Stye Ophthalmic Ointment	Oint, 55%/32%	PRN	For external use only, **not** for ocular use. Marketed to relieve some of the symptoms associated with a **hordeolum**

[a]Not for pregnant women or patients with renal failure, coagulopathy.
[b]For protocol refer to Cullom RD, Chang B, eds. The *Wills eye manual: office and emergency room diagnosis and treatment of eye disease*, 2nd ed. Philadelphia, JB Lippincott Co, 1994.
[c]*Arch Ophthalmol* 1990;108:689.

HOMEOPATHIC DRUGS

Note: The authors do not generally prescribe these remedies; however, the information is provided below.

Drug	Trade	Preparation	Usual dosage	Notes
N/A[a]	Optique	Soln	PRN	Preservative-free homeopathic drug for eye irritation from allergy, fatigue, pollution
N/A	Simalasan # 1	Soln	5–6 × day PRN	Homeopathic drug for dry eyes, preserved with Solusept
N/A	Simalasan #2	Soln	5–6 × day PRN	Homeopathic drug for allergic conjunctivitis, preserved with Solusept
succus cinarium maritima	SCM	Soln	BID	Homeopathic drug marketed to retard progression of cataracts

[a]N/A, not available.

Appendix 1. Topical Antibacterial Spectrum

	baci	ceph	CAM	cipro	erythro	gent	tetra/poly	norflox	polyB	poly/trimeth	sulfa	tobra	vanco
Gram+													
Staphylococcus aureus (MS)	+	+	+	+	i	+	+	+	o	+	+	+	+
Staphylococcus epidermidis	+	i	o	+	o	+	+	+	o	+	o	+	+
Streptococcus pyogenes	+	+	o	+	+	+	+	o	o	+	o	+	+
Streptococcus pneumoniae	+	+	+	+	+	+	+	+	o	+	+	+	+
Streptococcus viridans	+	o	o	+	+	o	+	o	o	+	+	o	+
Enterococcus faecalis	+	o	o	i	o	o	o	+	o	o	o	o	+
Bacillus cereus	o	o	+	o	+	+	i	+	o	o	o	+	+
Gram−													
Escherichia coli	o	+	+	+	o	+	+	+	+	+	+	+	o
Haemophilus influenzae	o	+	+	+	i	+	+	+	o	+	+	+	o
Klebsiella species	o	+	+	+	o	+	+	+	+	+	+	+	o

	baci	ceph	CAM	cipro	erythro	gent	tetra/poly	norflox	polyB	poly/trimeth	sulfa	tobra	vanco
Enterobacter species	o	o	+	+	o	+	o	+	+	+	+	+	+	o
Moraxella species	o	+	+	+	o	o	o	o	o	o	o	o	+	o
Neisseria species	+	+	+	+	+	o	o	o	o	o	i	+	+	i
Pseudomonas aeruginosa	o	o	+	+	o	o	o	o	i	i	i	i	i	o
Serratia marcescens	o	o	+	+	+	+	o	o	o	o	o	+	+	o
Aeromonas species	o	o	i	+	o	+	o	+	o	o	o	o	o	o
Acinetobacter species	+	o	o	+	o	+	o	i	i	o	o	+	+	o
Anaerobic														
Bacteroides fragilis	o	o	+	o	o	o	o	o	o	o	o	o	o	o
Propionibacterium acnes	o	o	o	o	i	o	o	i	o	o	o	o	o	+

+, sensitive; o, not sensitive; i, intermediate activity; baci, bacitracin; ceph, cephazolin; CAM, chloramphenicol; cipro, ciprofoxacin; erythro, erythromycin; gent, gentamicin; tetra/poly, tetracycline/polymyxin B; norflox, norfloxacin; polyB, polymyxin B; poly/trimeth, polymyxin B/trimethoprim; sulfa, sulfacetamide; tobra, tobramycin; vanco, vancomycin.
Table compiled from information in *Physicians' desk reference for ophthalmology*, 1996; Sanford JP, Gilbert DN, Sande, MA. *Sanford guide to antimicrobial therapy*. Dallas, Texas: Antimicrobial Therapy, Inc., 1995; Gilman AG, Rall TW, Nies AS, Taylor P. *Goodman and Gilman's The pharmacological basis of therapeutics*. Oxford: Pergamon Press, 1990; Murray PR, Baron EJ, Pfaller MA, Tenover FC, Yolken RH. *Manual of clinical microbiology*, 6th ed. Washington, DC: American Society for Microbiology Press, 1995.

Appendices

Appendix 2. Preparing Fortified Topical Antibiotics and Oral Acetafzolamide Solution

Preparing Fortified Topical Antibiotics[1]

Fortified Bacitracin

Add enough sterile water (without preservative) to 50,000 U of bacitracin dry powder to form 5 ml of solution. This provides a strength of 10,000 U per ml. Refrigerate. Expires after 7 days.

Fortified Cefazolin

Add enough sterile water (without preservative) to 500 mg of cefazolin dry powder to form 10 ml of solution. This provides a strength of 50 mg per ml. Refrigerate. Expires after 7 days.

Fortified Tobramycin (or Gentamicin)

With a syringe, inject 2 ml of tobramycin 40 mg per ml directly into a 5-ml bottle of tobramycin 0.3% ophthalmic solution (e.g.,

Tobrex). This gives a 7-ml solution of fortified tobramycin (approximately 15 mg per ml). Refrigerate. Expires after 14 days.

Fortified Vancomycin

Add enough sterile water (without preservative) to 500 mg of vancomycin dry powder to form 10 ml of solution. This provides a strength of 50 mg per ml. To achieve a 25 mg per ml concentration, take 5 ml of 50 mg per ml solution and add 5 ml of sterile water. Refrigerate. Expires after 4 days.

Preparing Oral Acetazolamide Solution

Dilute IV preparation in fruit juice such that one teaspoon (5 cc) contains correct unit dose (5 to 10 mg per kg per dose) (expensive) or prepare suspension with crushed pills and shake well. Expires after 5 days.

[1] Cullom RD, Chang B, eds. The Wills eye manual: office and emergency room diagnosis and treatment of Eye Disease, 2nd ed. Philadelphia: JB Lippincott Co, 1994:459.

Appendix 3. Antifungal Activity Spectrum

	Aspergillus	Blastomyces	Candida[a]	Coccidiodes	Cryptococcus	Fusarium	Histoplasma	Penicillium	Z Mucor
Amphotericin	x	x	x	x	x	x/—	x	x/—	x
Fluconazole	o	o	x	o	x	o	o	o	o
Flucytosine	o	o	x	o	x	o	o	o	o
Itraconazole	o	x	x	o	x/—	o	x	o	o
Ketoconazole	o	o	x	o	o	o	x	o	o
Miconazole	x	o	x	o	x	o	o	o	o
Natamycin	x	o	x	o	o	x	o	x	o

[a]*Candida* develops resistance quickly to flucytosine.

Note: Table represents *in vitro* sensitivities, which may or may not correlate with *in vivo* situations. Additionally, sensitivities will vary among institutions.

Information compiled from *Physicians' desk reference*, 50th ed. 1996.

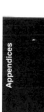

Appendices

Appendix 4. Renal Dosing for Selected Drugs

Creatinine clearance for men (140 − age [yr]) (body weight [kg])/72 (serum creatinine [mg/dl])
Creatinine clearance for women 0.85 × value for men

Acyclovir Dosing in Renal Failure[a]

Creatinine clearance (ml/min)	Percent of recommended dose	Dosing interval (hr)
≥50	100	8
25–50	100	12
10–25	100	24
<10	50	24

[a]Data from *Physicians' desk reference*, 51st ed. 1997.

Foscarnet Dosing in Renal Failure[a,b]

Creatinine clearance (ml/min/kg)	Resistant HSV (mg/kg)	CMV induction (mg/kg)
>1.4	40Q8hr	60Q8hr
>1.0–1.4	30Q8hr	45Q8hr
>0.8–1.0	35Q12hr	50Q12hr
>0.6–0.8	25Q12hr	40Q12hr
>0.5–0.6	40Q24hr	60Q24hr
≥0.4–0.5	35Q24hr	50Q24hr
<0.4	Not recommended	Not recommended

Creatinine clearance (ml/min/kg)	CMV maintenance [equiv. to 90 mg/kg/day (mg/kg)]	CMV maintenance [equiv. to 120 mg/kg/day (mg/kg)]
>1.4	90Q24hr	120Q24hr
>1.0–1.4	70Q24hr	90Q24hr
>0.8–1.0	50Q24hr	65Q24hr
>0.6–0.8	80Q48hr	105Q48hr
>0.5–0.6	60Q48hr	80Q48hr
≥0.4–0.5	50Q48hr	65Q48hr
<0.4	Not recommended	Not recommended

[a]Data from *Physicians' desk reference*, 51st ed. 1997.
[b]Delete body weight from calculation for foscarnet since creatinine clearance units are different (ml/min/kg). HSV, herpes simplex virus; CMV, cytomegalovirus.

Appendices

Intravenous Ganciclovir Dosing in Renal Failure[a]

Creatinine clearance (ml/min)	Induction dosage (mg/kg)	Maintenance dosage (mg/kg)
≥70	5.0Q12hr	5.0Q24hr
50–69	2.5Q12hr	2.5Q24hr
25–49	2.5Q24hr	1.25Q24hr
10–24	1.25Q24hr	0.625Q24hr
<10	1.25,3×/wk posthemodialysis	0.625, 3×/wk posthemodialysis

[a]Data from *Physicians' desk reference*, 51st ed. 1997.

Cidofovir Dosing in Renal Failure[a]

Creatinine clearance (ml/min)	Induction (once weekly for 2 wk) (mg/kg)	Maintenance (once every 2 wk) (mg/kg)
41–55	2.0	2.0
30–40	1.5	1.5
20–29	1.0	1.0
≤19	0.5	0.5

[a]Data from *Physicians' desk reference*, 51st ed. 1997.

Appendix 5. Glaucoma Medication Preservatives

Preservative	Drug	Trade
None	timolol maleate	Timoptic (dropettes)
Benzalkonium chloride	apraclonidine	Iopidine
	betaxolol	Betoptic, Betoptic-S
	brimonidine	Alphagan
	carbachol	Isopto Carbachol
	carteolol	Ocupress
	demecarium bromide	Humorsol
	dipivefrin	Propine
	dorzolamide	Trusopt
	epinephrine	Epifrin
	epinephrine/pilocarpine	E-Pilo
	latanaprost	Xalatan
	levobunolol	Betagan
	metipranolol	Optipranolol
	pilocarpine hydrochloride	Isopto Carpine, Pilocar, Pilostat, Pilopine HS gel
	timolol maleate	Timoptic
	timolol hemihydrate	Betimol
Benzododecinium bromide	timolol maleate	Timoptic XE
Chlorobutanol	echothiophate iodide	Phospholine Iodide
	pilocarpine nitrate	Pilagan
Ethylene/vinyl acetate membrane	pilocarpine hydrochloride	Ocusert Pilo 20, Ocusert Pilo 40

Product Index

Subject Index

Subject
Index